MW00568013

MILADY'S
Theory and Practice of Therapeutic Massage Workbook

To be used with

MILADY'S Theory and Practice of Therapeutic Massage
Second Edition

Mark F. Beck

Milady Publishing Company
(A Division of Delmar Publishers Inc.)
3 Columbia Circle, Box 12519
Albany, New York 12212-2519

NOTICE TO THE READER

Publisher does not warrant or guarantee any of the products described herein or perform any independent analysis in connection with any of the product information contained herein. Publisher does not assume, and expressly disclaims, any obligation to obtain and include information other than that provided to it by the manufacturer.

The reader is expressly warned to consider and adopt all safety precautions that might be indicated by the activities described herein and to avoid all potential hazards. By following the instructions contained herein, the reader willingly assumes all risks in connection with such instructions.

The publisher makes no representations or warranties of any kind, including but not limited to, the warranties of fitness for particular purpose or merchantability, nor are any such representations implied with respect to the material set forth herein, and the publisher takes no responsibility with respect to such material. The publisher shall not be liable for any special, consequential or exemplary damages resulting, in whole or in part, from the readers' use of, or reliance upon, this material.

Delmar Publishers' Online Services
To access Delmar on the World Wide Web, point your browser to:
http://www.delmar.com/delmar.html
To access through Gopher: gopher://gopher.delmar.com
(Delmar Online is part of "thomson.com", an Internet site with information on
more than 30 publishers of the International Thomson Publishing organization.)
For information on our products and services:
email: info@delmar.com
or call 800-347-7707

For information address:
Milady Publishing Company
(A Division of Delmar Publishers Inc.)
3 Columbia Circle, Box 12519
Albany, NY 12212-2519

Copyright © 1994
Milady Publishing Company
(A Division of Delmar Publishers Inc.)

All rights reserved. No part of this work covered by the copyright hereon may be reproduced or used in any form or by any means—graphic, electronic, or mechanical, including photocopying, recording, taping, or information storage and retrieval systems—without written permission of the publisher.

Printed in the United States of America
Printed and published simultaneously in Canada

2 3 4 5 6 7 8 9 10 XXX 00 99 98 97 96 95

Library of Congress Catalog Card Number: 93–28234

ISBN: 1–56253–216–2

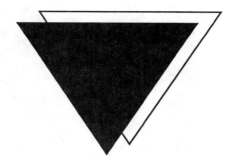

Contents

How to Use This Workbook

Milady's Theory and Practice of Therapeutic Massage Workbook has been written to meet the needs, interests, and abilities of students receiving training in therapeutic massage.

This workbook should be used together with *Milady's Theory and Practice of Therapeutic Massage Workbook*. This book directly follows the information found in the student textbook.

Students are to answer each item in this workbook with a pencil after consulting their textbook for correct information. Items can be corrected and/or rated during class or individual discussions, or on an independent study basis.

Various tests are included to emphasize essential facts found in the textbook and to measure the student's progress. "Word Reviews" are listed for each chapter. They are to be used as study guides, for class discussions, or for the teacher to assign groups of words to be used by the student in creative essays.

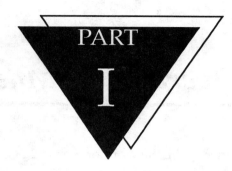

The History and Advancement of Therapeutic Massage

Historical Overview of Massage

Completion: In the space provided write the word or words that correctly complete each statement.

1. When was the term *massage* first used in American or European literature to denote using the hands to apply manipulations to the soft tissues?

   _____.

2. Two terms the Chinese use for systems of massage are _____ and _____.

3. There is documentation that the Chinese have practiced massage since _____.

4. The Japanese style of massage that uses finger pressure is _____.

5. A sacred book of the Hindus written around 1800 B.C. is the _____.

6. The Hindu practice of bathing and massage that included kneading the extremities, tapotement, frictioning, anointing with perfumes, and cracking the joints of the fingers, toes, and the neck was known as _____.

7. The _____ is a code of ethics for physicians and those about to receive medical degrees that binds them to honor their teachers, do their best to maintain the health of their patients, honor their patients' secrets, and prescribe no harmful treatment or drug.

8. The word Hippocrates used to denote the art of rubbing upward not downward is _____.

Matching: Match the name with the best description. Write the letter of that name in the space provided.

A. Aesculapius
B. Avicenna
C. Celcus
D. Dr. James H. Cyriax
E. Elizabeth Dicke
F. Maria Ebner

G. Dr. Douglas O. Graham
H. Hippocrates
I. Albert J. Hoffa
J. Per Henrik Ling
K. Dr. Johann G. Mezger
L. Ambroise Pare

M. Mathias Roth
N. Charles Fayette Taylor
O. George Henry Taylor
P. Emil Vodder

_____ 1. Popularized the use of the word *massage* in America

___K___ 2. Credited with popularizing the terms *effleurage, petrissage, tappotments,* and *friction*

_____ 3. The Greek physician later worshipped as the "god of medicine" who founded the first gymnasium

___H___ 4. The Greek physician who became known as the father of medicine

_____ 5. The name of the Roman physician who wrote *De Medicina*

_____ 6. The Persian philosopher/physician who authored the *Canon of Medicine*

_____ 7. The French barber/surgeon who was one of the founders of modern surgery and who described in his publications the positive effects of massage in the healing process

_____ 8. Known as "the father of physical therapy;" developed a system of movements he called "medical gymnastics"

_____ 9. The English physician who published the first book in English on the Swedish movements

_____ 10. Established the first institute in England to teach Swedish movement gymnastics

_____ 11. The New York physician who introduced the Swedish movements to the United States in 1858

_____ 12. Physician's brother who published the first American textbook on the Swedish movement

_____ 13. Acknowledged by many of the authors of his day as "the founder of scientific massage"

_____ 14. Considered by some to be "the father of Swedish massage in the United States"

_____ 15. The distinguished German physician who published *Technik Der Massage*

_____ 16. The Austrian who developed a method of lymph massage

_____ 17. Developed Bindegewebsmassage

_____ 18. Popularized Bindegewebsmassage in England

_____ 19. The English orthopedic physician credited with popularizing deep transverse friction massage

Matching: Match the term with the best description. Write the letter of the appropriate term in the space provided.

A. acupressure   C. Rolfing   E. sports massage

B. reflexology   D. Shiatsu   F. Swedish massage

_____ 1. Based on the western concepts of anatomy and physiology, and employs effleurage, petrissage, vibration, friction, and tappotement

_____ 2. Based in the Traditional Oriental Medical principles for assessing and treating the physical and energetic body order to regulate Chi (the life force energy)

_____ 3. A finger pressure method based on the Oriental concept that the body has a series of energy (tsubo) points

_____ 4. A method of massage especially designed to prepare an athlete for an upcoming event and to aid in the body's regenerative and restorative capacities following a rigorous workout or competition

_____ 5. Developed out of the technique of structural integration, it aligns the major body segments through manipulation of the fascia or the connective tissue

_____ 6. A method based on the idea that stimulation of particular points on the surface of the body has an effect on other areas or organs of the body

Requirements for the Practice of Therapeutic Massage

Short Answer: In the space provided, write a short answer to the following questions.

1. What is meant by "the scope of practice?"

   _____

   _____

2. In states that have massage licensing, how is the scope of practice defined?

   _____

   _____

3. In the United States what jurisdiction might oversee regulations for massage?

   _____

   _____

4. What is the major reason for licensing massage therapists?

   _____

5. What is the role of national or state regulatory boards?

   _____

6. Besides massage licensing laws and ordinances, what other laws must be abided when operating a massage business?

   _____

True or False: If the following statements are true, write *true* in the space provided. If they are false, write *false*.

_____ 1. If a massage therapist is nationally certified, they can practice anywhere in the United States.

_____ 2. Reciprocity means that if a massage therapist has a license in one place he or she can practice anywhere.

_____ 3. In a state that has massage licensing, if a licensed nurse or chiropractor wants to practice massage, they must obtain a massage license.

_____ 4. The scope of practice for massage is clearly defined by national standards.

Short Answer: Of the following statements, put a check mark in front of the ones that may be grounds for revoking, canceling, or suspending a massage license.

_____ 1. Having been convicted of a felony

_____ 2. Being guilty of fraudulent or deceptive advertising

_____ 3. Being engaged currently or previously in any act of prostitution

_____ 4. Practicing under a false or assumed name

_____ 5. Being accused of making sexual advances or attempting sexual acts during the course of a massage

_____ 6. Prescribing drugs or medicines (unless you are a licensed physician)

_____ 7. Charging extremely high fees for the services provided

_____ 8. Being addicted to narcotics, alcohol, or like substances that interfere with the performance of duties

_____ 9. Being guilty of fraud or deceit in obtaining a license

_____ 10. Selling nutritional products or other non-massage related items

_____ 11. Being willfully negligent in the practice of massage so as to endanger the health of a client

Completion: In the spaces provided, write the word or words that correctly complete each statement.

1. A _____ is issued by a state or municipal regulating agency as a requirement for conducting a business or practicing a trade or profession.

2. A document that is awarded in recognition of an accomplishment or for achieving or maintaining some kind of standard is a _____.

Professional Ethics for Massage Practitioners

Completion: In the spaces provided, write the word or words from the list below that correctly complete each statement.

confidential	fairness	a satisfied customer
courtesy	honest	sexual
ethics	professional	tactful

1. The standards and philosophy of human conduct or code of morals of an individual, group, or profession is known as _____.

2. One of the best forms of advertising in a personal service business is

   _____.

3. A person engaged in an avocation or occupation requiring advanced training to gain knowledge and skills is considered a _____.

4. All clients should be treated with _____ and _____.

5. All communications with clients should be _____ and _____.

6. Be respectful of the therapeutic relationship and maintain appropriate _____ boundaries.

7. In order to deal with a client who is overly critical, finds fault, and is hard to please, the therapist must be _____.

Short Answer: In the space provided, write a short answer to the following question.

1. List nine attributes that are helpful for developing good human relations between therapist and client.

    a. _____

    b. _____

    c. _____

    d. _____

    e. _____

    f. _____

    g. _____

    h. _____

    i. _____

2. Name three ways to stay current regarding the massage profession.

    a. _____

    b. _____

    c. _____

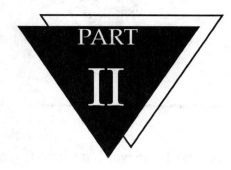

Human Anatomy and Physiology

Overview

Completion: In the space provided, write the word or words that correctly complete each statement.

1. The study of the gross structure of the body or the study of an organism and the interrelations of its parts is _____.

2. The science and study of the vital processes, mechanisms, and functions of an organ or system of organs is _____.

3. The branch of biology concerned with the microscopic structure of tissues of a living organism is _____.

4. The study of the structural and functional changes caused by disease is _____.

5. The delicate physiological balance the body strives to maintain in its internal environment is _____.

6. The abnormal and unhealthy state of all or part of the body where it is not capable of carrying on its normal function is _____.

7. A _____ of a disease is perceived by the victim while a _____ of a disease is observable by another individual.

Key Choices: Massage may have a direct, an indirect, or a reflex effect on various functions of the body. Put the appropriate letter in the space provided for each of the following phrases.

D = Direct effect

I = Indirect effect

R = Reflex effect

_____ 1. Increased circulation to the muscles and internal organs

_____ 2. Stretching of muscles tissue

_____ 3. Slower, deeper breathing

_____ 4. Loosening of adhesions and scar tissue

_____ 5. Reduced heart rate

_____ 6. Reduced blood pressure

_____ 7. Increased local circulation of venous blood

_____ 8. General relaxation of tense muscles

Key Choices: Most diseases have signs and/or symptoms. Put the appropriate letter in the space provided for each of the following phrases.

X = Disease symptom

O = Sign of disease

_____ 1. nausea

_____ 2. abnormal skin color

_____ 3. pain

_____ 4. chills

_____ 5. elevated pulse

_____ 6. severe itching

_____ 7. abdominal cramps

_____ 8. fever

_____ 9. dizziness

_____ 10. skin ulcers

Completion: In the space provided, write the word or words that correctly complete each statement.

1. Two hormones that are secreted by the adrenal glands are _____ and _____.

2. The protective body sensation that warns of tissue damage or destruction is _____.

3. The two reactions to pain are _____ and _____.

4. Inhibited blood flow to an area of the body is known as _____.

5. A syndrome that often starts as a simple muscle spasm that is complicated by muscle splinting and constricted circulation is the _____.

6. Much of the discomfort in the condition of the previous question is from _____.

7. Psychologically, skillfully applied therapeutic massage helps to reduce pain by relieving _____ and _____.

8. In a pain-spasm-pain cycle, pain is intensified because of _____.

9. Therapeutic massage on contracted ischemic tissue relieves _____ and restores _____.

10. Pain is an indication of _____ or _____.

11. Generally, the more severe the pain the more severe the _____.

12. Bacteria, viruses, fungi, and protozoa are _____.

13. If they enter the body in large enough numbers to multiply and become capable of destroying health tissue they cause _____.

14. If these organisms are confined to a small area, the condition is considered a _____ but if they spread through the body, the condition is termed a _____.

15. When tissue is damaged from invading organisms or physical injury, substances are released that cause _____.

16. The four signs and symptoms of inflammation are _____ and _____.

17. An elevated body temperature that accompanies infectious diseases is a _____.

18. The fibrous connective tissue formed as a wound heals is _____. Connective tissue fibers are produced in healing tissue by _____.

Short Answer: In the space provided, write a short answer to the following questions.

1. List six possible direct causes of disease.

   a. _____

   b. _____

   c. _____

   d. _____

   e. _____

   f. _____

2. Stress is most notably associated with the adrenal glands and their secretion of the "fight or flight" hormones. Briefly describe what happens to the following body functions during the "fight or flight" reaction.

   1. Muscle tone _____

   2. Blood pressure _____

   3. Digestion _____

   4. Circulation to skeletal muscles _____

   5. Circulation to digestive organs _____

   6. Red blood cells _____

3. Different types of tissue heal at different rates. Number the following from 1 to 5 according to how fast they mend: 1 is the fastest, 5 is the slowest.

   _____ nerve tissue

   _____ bone

   _____ skin

   _____ muscle

   _____ ligament

Completion: In the space provided, write the word or words that correctly complete each statement.

1. Physiologically, skillfully applied therapeutic massage helps to reduce pain by providing _____

   _____.

2. If massage increases the overall intensity of the pain, the therapist should _____

   _____.

3. A wellness-oriented individual attempts to maintain a balance between _____

   _____ and _____.

4. In medical terminology, compound words are constructed of _____

   _____ and _____.

Matching: Match the term in the first column with the meaning in the second column by placing the correct letter in the space provided.

WORD ROOTS I

_____ 1. arth(ro)   A. lung

_____ 2. chondr/o   B. tissue

_____ 3. cyt   C. joint

_____ 4. hem   D. nerve

_____ 5. hist   E. cell

_____ 6. my(o)   F. heat

_____ 7. neur(o)   G. blood

_____ 8. oss, ost(e)   H. vessel

_____ 9. phleb   I. bone

_____ 10. pulmo   J. cartilage

_____ 11. therm   K. vein

_____ 12. vas   L. muscle

WORD ROOTS II

_____	1. brachi	A. head
_____	2. cardi	B. kidney
_____	3. cephal	C. foot
_____	4. derm	D. stomach
_____	5. gastr/o	E. arm
_____	6. gyn	F. woman
_____	7. hepat	G. skin
_____	8. labi	H. lung
_____	9. nephr(o)	I. liver
_____	10. ocul	J. heart
_____	11. pneum	K. eye
_____	12. pod	L. lip

PREFIXES I

_____	1. ab-	A. beyond, outside of, in addition
_____	2. ad-	B. against
_____	3. ant-	C. against, counter to
_____	4. ante-	D. away from
_____	5. bio-	E. inside
_____	6. contra-	F. above, in addition
_____	7. ex-	G. before
_____	8. infra-	H. out of
_____	9. extra-	I. to, toward
_____	10. intra-	J. beneath
_____	11. sub-	K. under, below
_____	12. super-	L. life

PREFIXES II

_____	1. ect-	A. under, below
_____	2. end-(o)	B. one, single
_____	3. epi-	C. inside, within
_____	4. hyper-	D. around
_____	5. hypo-	E. stupor, numbness
_____	6. mega-	F. upon, over, in addition
_____	7. micr-(o)	G. large, extreme
_____	8. mon-(o)	H. outside, without
_____	9. narc-	I. pertaining to disease
_____	10. path-	J. small
_____	11. peri-	K. false
_____	12. pseud-(o)	L. above, extreme

PREFIXES III

_____	1. hemi-	A. many, much
_____	2. hetero-	B. middle, midline
_____	3. hom-	C. the other
_____	4. medi-	D. together, along with
_____	5. multi-	E. four
_____	6. para-	F. single, one
_____	7. poly-	G. common, same
_____	8. quad-	H. many, multiple
_____	9. retro-	I. half
_____	10. syn-	J. three
_____	11. tri-	K. next to, resembling, beside
_____	12. uni-	L. backward

SUFFIXES

_____	1. -ase	A. diseased
_____	2. -algia	B. study of, science of
_____	3. -ectomy	C. forming an opening
_____	4. -graph	D. surgical removal of body part
_____	5. -ia	E. denoting an enzyme
_____	6. -itis	F. tumor
_____	7. -ology	G. write, draw, record
_____	8. -oma	H. morbid fear of
_____	9. -ostomy	I. excision, cutting into
_____	10. -otomy	J. painful condition
_____	11. -pathic	K. inflammation
_____	12. -phobia	L. a noun ending of a condition

Word Review: The student is encouraged to write down the meaning of each of the following words. The list can be used as a study guide for this unit.

adrenaline	homeostasis	pain-spasm-pain cycle
anatomy	infection	pathology
cortisol	inflammation	physiology
disease	ischemia	sign of disease
fever	ischemic pain	stress
fight or flight	medical terminology	symptom
histology	microorganisms	wellness

Human Anatomy and Physiology

Histology

Completion: In the space provided, write the word or words that correctly complete each statement.

1. The submicroscopic particles that make up all substances are called _____.

2. These are arranged in specific patterns and structures called _____.

3. In the human organism, the basic unit of structure and function is the _____.

4. These are organized into layers or groups called _____.

5. Groups of these form complex structures that perform certain functions. These structures are called _____ and are arranged in _____.

6. All living matter is composed of a colorless, jellylike substance called _____.

7. The cytoplasm contains a network of various membranes called _____ which perform specific functions necessary for cell survival.

8. Cell reproduction is controlled by the _____ and the _____.

9. During the early developmental stages of an organism, the repeated division of the ovum results in many specialized cells that differ from one another in composition and function. This process is _____.

10. In the human organism as a cell matures and is nourished, it grows in size and eventually divides into two smaller daughterlike cells. This form of cell division is called _____.

Short Answer: In the space provided, write a short answer to the following questions.

1. Name four ways in which cells differ from one another.

   a. _____ c. _____

   b. _____ d. _____

2. Name the four principle parts of a cell.

   a. _____ c. _____

   b. _____ d. _____

Identification: Identify the indicated structures in Figure 5.1. Write the correct letter next to the appropriate name in the space provided.

_____ 1. cell membrane

_____ 2. chromatin

_____ 3. smooth endoplasmic reticulum

_____ 4. Golgi apparatus

_____ 5. lysosome

_____ 6. pinocytic vessel

_____ 7. mitochondrion

_____ 8. nucleolus

_____ 9. nucleus

_____ 10. ribosomes

_____ 11. vacuole

_____ 12. rough endoplasmic
reticulum

_____ 13. cytoplasm

Matching: Match each term with its associated function. Write the letter of the function in the space provided.

A. cell membrane

B. centrosome

C. chromatin

D. endoplasmic reticulum

E. fibrils

F. Golgi apparatus

G. lysosome

H. microtubules

I. mitochondria

J. nuclear membrane

K. nucleolus

L. nucleus

M. ribosome

N. vacuole

_____ 1. converts and releases energy for cell operation

_____ 2. contains cellular material and transports materials between the inside and outside of the cell

_____ 3. produce lipids or proteins for cell utilization and transport

_____ 4. supervises all cell activity

_____ 5. synthesizes carbohydrates and holds protein for secretion

_____ 6. Involved in the rapid introduction or ejection of substances

_____ 7. divides and moves to opposite poles of the cell during mitosis

_____ 8. controls passage of substances between the nucleus and cytoplasm

_____ 9. composed of RNA and protein molecules that synthesize proteins

_____ 10. fibers of protein and DNA that contain the genes

Short Answer: The five phases of cell division are listed below. Number the phases from 1 to 5 to indicate the correct order in which they occur.

_____ metaphase   _____ interphase   _____ anaphase

_____ telophase   _____ prophase

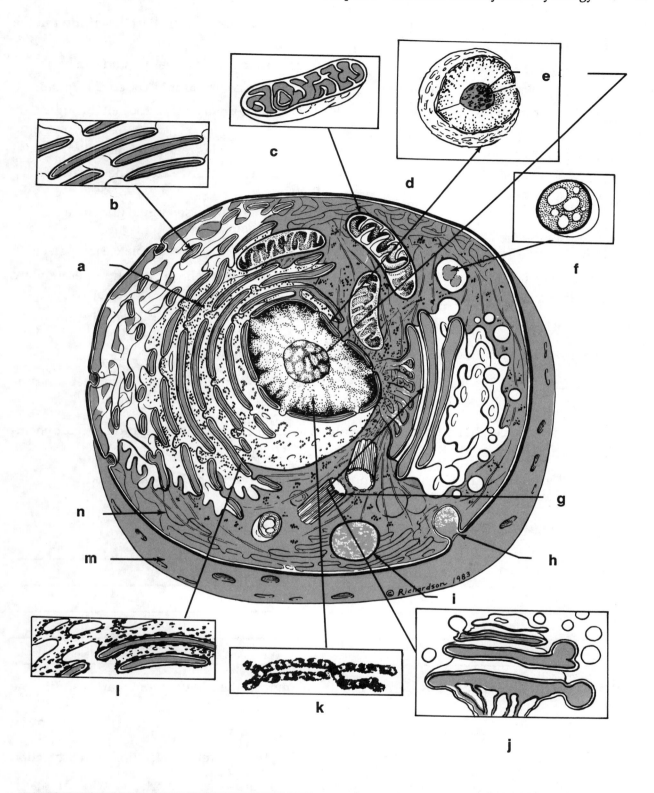

Fig. 5.1   Structure of a typical animal cell.

Matching: Match the term with the best description. Write the letter of the best description in the space provided.

_____ 1. metaphase

_____ 2. telophase

_____ 3. interphase

_____ 4. prophase

_____ 5. anaphase

A. Chromosomes become larger and can be seen as two coiled strands called chromatids.

B. This is the normal state of the cell during growth.

C. Cytoplasm divides into two cells.

D. Chromosomes arrange along the equatorial plane.

E. The chromatids are separated and are again called chromosomes.

Completion: In the space provided, write the word or words that correctly complete each statement.

1. The chemical reactions within a cell that transform food for cell growth and operation are broadly termed _____.

2. Two phases of metabolism are _____ and _____.

3. The process of building up larger molecules from smaller ones is _____.

4. The process of breaking down larger substances or molecules into smaller ones is _____.

5. Protein substances that act as organic catalysts to initiate, accelerate, or control specific chemical reactions in the metabolic process are called _____.

6. Collections of similar cells that carry out specific functions of the body are called _____.

Short Answer: List the five main categories of tissues in the space provided.

1. _____

2. _____

3. _____

4. _____

5. _____

Identification: In the space provided, write the name of the tissue type that best fits the description.

_____ 1. represented by blood and lymph

_____ 2. functions in the process of absorption, excretion, secretion, and protection

_____ 3. binds structures together and serves as a framework

_____ 4. acts as a channel for the transmission of messages

_____ 5. forms the skin, the covering of the organs, and the inner lining of all the hollow organs

_____ 6. carries nutrients to the cells and carries away waste products

_____ 7. deep fascia, superficial fascia

_____ 8. initiates, controls, and coordinates the body's adaptation to its surroundings

_____ 9. contracts and causes movement

_____ 10. always has a free surface that is exposed to outside influences

_____ 11. responsible for the movement of food through the digestive tract, the constriction of blood vessels, and the emptying of the bladder

_____ 12. bones, cartilage and ligaments

_____ 13. cells classified by shape as squamous, cuboidal, and columnar

_____ 14. collects into the lymphatic vessels along with metabolic waste and toxins

_____ 15. provides support and protection

_____ 16. covers all the surfaces of the body

_____ 17. responsible for pumping blood through the heart into the blood vessels

_____ 18. composed of neurons

_____ 19. circulates throughout the body

_____ 20. makes up the major tissue of the glands

_____ 21. responsible for facial expression, speaking, and other voluntary movements

Completion: In the space provided, write the word or words that correctly complete each statement.

1. Two categories of membranes are _____ membranes and _____ _____ membranes.

2. _____ produce a thick, sticky substance that acts as a protectant and lubricant.

3. _____ produce a more watery, lubricating substance that lines the body cavities and sometimes forms the outermost surface of the organs contained in those cavities.

4. Three major serous membranes are the _____ that encase the lungs, the _____ around the heart, and the _____ that lines the abdominal cavity.

Short Answer: In the space provided, write a short answer to the question.

1. List three types of fascial membranes.

    a. _____

    b. _____

    c. _____

2. Name three types of skeletal membrane and state where it is found.

   a. _____

   b. _____

   c. _____

Matching: Match the term with the best description. Write the letter of the best description in the space provided.

_____ 1. elastic cartilage

_____ 2. areolar tissue

_____ 3. osseous tissue

_____ 4. adipose tissue

_____ 5. ligaments

_____ 6. fibrocartilage

_____ 7. fibrous connective tissue

_____ 8. tendons

_____ 9. hyaline cartilage

A. impregnated with mineral salts, chiefly calcium phosphate and calcium carbonate

B. found between the vertebrae and in the pubic symphysis

C. found in the external ear and the larynx

D. found on the end of bones and in movable joints.

E. fibrous bands that connect bones to bones

F. composed of collagen and elastic fibers that are closely arranged

G. cords or bands that serve to attach muscle to bone

H. binds the skin to the underlying tissues and fills the spaces between the muscles

I. has an abundance of fat-containing cells

Completion: In the space provided, write the word or words that correctly complete each statement.

1. The three types of muscle tissue are _____ and _____.

2. _____ are usually attached to bone or other muscle by way of tendons and can be controlled by conscious effort.

3. Because these muscles have alternating light and dark crossmarkings, they are called _____.

4. Muscle tissue found in the hollow organs of the stomach, small intestine, colon, bladder, and the blood vessels does not have the cross markings and is called _____ or _____ muscle.

5. _____ is found only in the heart.

Word Review: The student is encouraged to write down the meaning of each of the following words. The list can be used as a study guide for this unit.

adipose tissue	fibrocartilage	perichondrium
amitosis	fibrous connective tissue	periosteum
anabolism	enzymes	physiology
anaphase	epithelial membranes	prophase
anatomy	epithelial tissue	protoplasm
areolar tissue	fascia	reticular tissue
atoms	histology	serous membranes
cardiac muscle tissue	hyaline cartilage	skeletal muscle
catabolism	interphase	smooth muscle
cell	ligaments	squamous
cell membrane	metaphase	striated muscles
cellular metabolism	mitosis	superficial fascia
centrosome	molecules	synovial membrane
columnar	mucous membranes	telophase
connective tissue membranes	nerve tissue	tendons
cuboidal	neurons	tissues
cytoplasm	nucleus	voluntary muscles
cytoplasmic organelles	organ system	
differentiation	organs	

Organization of the Human Body

Completion: In the space provided, write the word or words that correctly complete each statement.

1. In the anatomic position, the body _____ with the palms of the hands facing _____.

2. Anatomists divide the body with three imaginary planes called the _____, the _____, and the _____ planes.

3. The _____ divides the body into left and right parts by an imaginary line running vertically down the body.

4. The _____ is an imaginary line that divides the body into the anterior [front] or ventral half of the body and the posterior [back] or dorsal half of the body.

5. The _____ is an imaginary line that divides the body horizontally into an upper and lower portion.

6. _____ refers to the plane that divides the body or an organ into right and left halves.

Matching: Match the term with the best description. Write the letter of the best description in the space provided.

_____ 1. cranial or superior aspect
_____ 2. caudal or inferior aspect
_____ 3. anterior or ventral aspect
_____ 4. posterior or dorsal aspect
_____ 5. transverse plane
_____ 6. sagittal plane
_____ 7. coronal plane
_____ 8. medial aspect
_____ 9. lateral aspect
_____ 10. distal aspect
_____ 11. proximal

A. situated in front of
B. situated farther from the crown of the head
C. farthest point from the origin of a structure or point of attachment
D. situated in back of
E. on the side, farther from the midline
F. nearest the origin of a structure or point of attachment
G. situated toward the crown of the head
H. dividing the body into right and left sides
I. the frontal plane dividing it into front and back halves
J. pertaining to the middle or nearer to the midline
K. a plane through a body part perpendicular to the axis

Identification: Figure 5.2 is a diagram of the various body cavities. Identify the indicated structures and write the correct names in the space provided.

1. _____

2. _____

3. _____

4. _____

5. _____

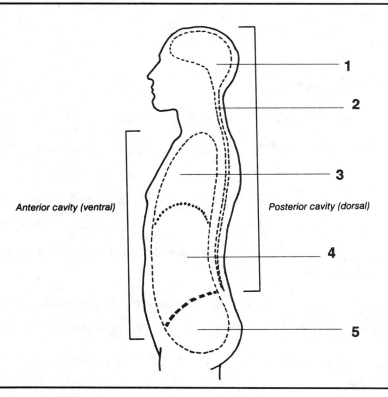

Fig. 5.2 Body cavities.

Matching: Match the term with the best description. Write the letter of the best description in the space provided.

_____ 1. hypogastric

_____ 2. inguinal

_____ 3. temporal

_____ 4. scapular

_____ 5. frontal

_____ 6. brachial

_____ 7. cervical

_____ 8. deltoid

_____ 9. umbilical

_____ 10. epigastric

_____ 11. lumbar

_____ 12. gluteal

_____ 13. patellar

_____ 14. popliteal

_____ 15. pectoral

_____ 16. parietal

_____ 17. axillary

_____ 18. femoral

_____ 19. mastoid

_____ 20. hypochondrium

A. region of the temples

B. region of the neck

C. region of the shoulder joint and deltoid muscle

D. region of the armpit

E. region between the elbow and shoulder

F. region of the abdomen lateral to the epigastric region

G. region of the navel

H. region inferior to the umbilical region

I. region of the kneecap

J. region of the thigh

K. region of the groin

L. region of the lower back

M. region of the abdomen

N. region of the breast and chest

O. region of the head, posterior to the frontal region and anterior to the occipital region

P. region of the temporal bone behind the ear

Q. region of muscles of the buttocks

R. region of the back of the shoulder or shoulder blade

S. an area behind the knee joint

T. region of the forehead

Identification: Identify the indicated anatomical areas in Figure 5.3 and 5.4. Write the correct letter next to the appropriate names in the space provided.

_____ 1. axillary

_____ 2. brachial

_____ 3. cervical

_____ 4. epigastric

_____ 5. femoral

_____ 6. frontal

_____ 7. gluteal

_____ 8. hypochondriac

_____ 9. hypogastric

_____ 10. inguinal

_____ 11. lumbar

_____ 12. occipital

_____ 13. parietal

_____ 14. patellar

_____ 15. pectoral

_____ 16. popliteal

_____ 17. sacral

_____ 18. scapular

_____ 19. temporal

_____ 20. umbilical

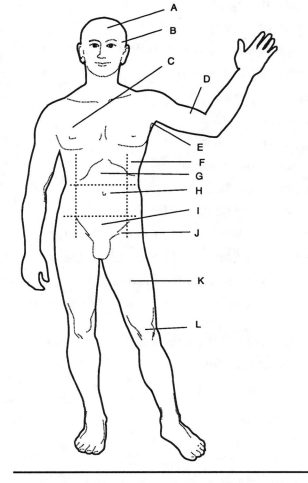

Fig. 5.3 Regions of the body, anterior view.

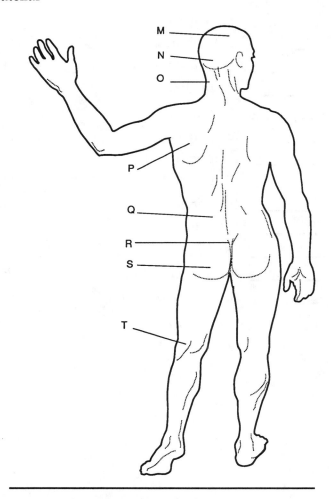

Fig. 5.4 Regions of the body, posterior view.

Completion: In the space provided, write the word or words that correctly complete each statement.

1. The dorsal cavities include the _____ cavity and the _____ cavity.

2. The ventral cavities are the _____ cavity and _____ cavities.

3. The liver, stomach, spleen, pancreas, and small and large intestines are located in the _____ cavity.

4. The _____ contains the bladder, rectum, and some of the reproductive organs.

5. The four main anatomical parts of the body are _____.

6. Body structures containing two or more different tissues that combine to perform a definite function are called _____.

7. When a number of organs work together to perform a bodily function, they comprise an _____.

Short Answer: List ten organ systems.

1. _____

2. _____

3. _____

4. _____

5. _____

6. _____

7. _____

8. _____

9. _____

10. _____

Identification: In the space provided write the name of the related major body system.

_____ 1. carries oxygen and nutrients to all parts of the body

_____ 2. is damaged with a scratch or burn

_____ 3. provides a rigid structure and attachment for muscles

_____ 4. breaks down food into absorbable particles

_____ 5. includes pituitary, thyroid, and ovaries

_____ 6. produces heat and movement

_____ 7. removes uric acid from the system

_____ 8. provides for continuation of the species

_____ 9. allows for the absorption of oxygen into the body

_____ 10. includes the liver, lungs, kidneys, and colon

_____ 11. provides information as to where we are in the environment

_____ 12. produces hormones

Word Review: The student is encouraged to write down the meaning of each of the following words. This list can be used as a study guide for this unit.

abdominal cavities	hormones	proximal
anatomic position	inferior	respiratory system
anterior	integumentary system	sagittal plane
circulatory system	lateral	skeletal system
coronal plane	lymph system	superior
cranial cavity	medial	thoracic cavity
digestive system	muscular system	transverse plane
distal	organ system	ventral cavities
dorsal cavities	nervous system	vertebral cavity
endocrine system	pelvic cavity	
excretory system	posterior	

System One: The Integumentary System—The Skin

Short Answer: List six functions of the skin.

1. _____
2. _____
3. _____
4. _____
5. _____
6. _____

Identification: Figure 5.5 shows a cross section of skin. Identify the indicated structures and write the correct letter next to the appropriate names in the space provided.

_____ 1. arrector pili muscle

_____ 2. dermis

_____ 3. epidermis

_____ 4. hair root

_____ 5. adipose

_____ 6. papilla of hair

_____ 7. sebaceous duct

_____ 8. capillaries

_____ 9. pacinian corpuscle

_____ 10. vein

_____ 11. hair shaft

_____ 12. Meissner corpuscle

_____ 13. reticular fibers

_____ 14. sebaceous gland

_____ 15. stratum corneum

_____ 16. stratum germinativum

_____ 17. stratum granulosum

_____ 18. subcutaneous tissue

_____ 19. papillary layer of dermis

_____ 20. sudoriferous gland

_____ 21. stratum lucidum

_____ 22. stratum spinosum

_____ 23. artery

_____ 24. epidermic scales

_____ 25. ruffian receptor

_____ 26. nerve

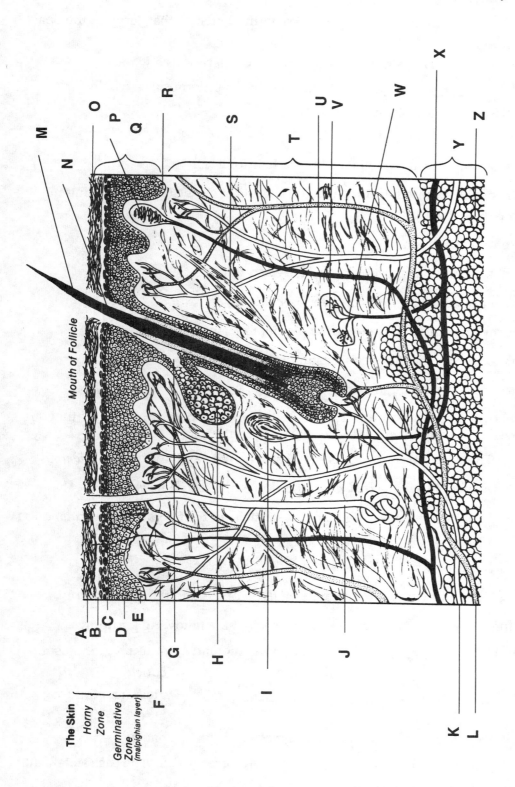

Fig. 5.5   The integumentary system (showing skin and hair).

Matching: Match the term with the best description. Write the letter of that term in the space provided.

A. papillary layer   D. stratum granulosum   G. dermis as a whole

B. reticular layer   E. malpighian layer   H. epidermis as a whole

C. subcutaneous tissue   F. stratum germinativum

_____ 1. the deepest layer of the epidermis

_____ 2. contains fat cells, sweat and oil glands, and hair follicles

_____ 3. contains conelike projections made of fine strands of elastic tissue extending upward into the epidermis

_____ 4. site of keratin formation

_____ 5. contains blood and lymph vessels, and nerve endings

_____ 6. serves as a protective cushion for the upper skin layers

_____ 7. contains melanocytes that produce the pigment melanin

_____ 8. contains collagen, reticulum, and elastin fibers

_____ 9. consists of cells containing melanin

True or False: If the following statements are true, write *true* in the space provided. If they are false, replace the italicized word with one that makes the statement true.

_____ 1. There is a fine network of blood and lymph capillaries in the *epidermis*.

_____ 2. As people age the *collagen* of the skin tends to lose its elasticity.

_____ 3. Pliability of the skin depends on elasticity of the fibers in the *subcutaneous layer*.

_____ 4. Healthy skin possesses a slightly *acid* reaction.

_____ 5. The color of the skin depends on *the thickness* and the blood supply.

Short Answer: Underline the term that does not belong in each of the following groupings.

stratum germinativum	_____	stratum malpighian	stratum granulosum
melanin	_____	keratin	cuticle
pacinian corpuscle	ruffian receptor	_____	meissner corpuscle
scar	_____	crust	fissure
_____	leucoderma	lentigines	naevus

Completion: In the space provided, write the word or words that correctly complete each statement.

1. There are two clearly defined divisions of the skin. The outer layer is the _____ and the inner layer is the _____.

2. There are two kinds of duct glands in the skin. _____ produce sweat and _____ glands produce oil.

3. Sweat glands are under the control of the _____ nervous system.

4. Two appendages of the skin are _____ and _____.

5. The appendages of the skin referred to in the previous question are composed of _____ _____.

6. The _____ muscle is connected to the base of the hair follicle.

7. When the muscle referred to in the previous question contracts, it results in a reaction commonly called _____.

8. A structural change in the tissues caused by injury or disease is a _____.

9. A structural change in the tissues that develop in the later stages of disease are called _____.

10. Small masses of hardened, discolored sebum that appear most frequently on the face, shoulders, chest, and back are called _____.

Matching: Match the term with the best description. Write the letter of that term in the space provided.

_____ 1. scar
_____ 2. macule
_____ 3. pustule
_____ 4. scale
_____ 5. tumor
_____ 6. vesicle
_____ 7. bulla
_____ 8. ulcer
_____ 9. wheal
_____ 10. papule
_____ 11. crust
_____ 12. fissure

A. an accumulation of epidermal flakes such as excessive dandruff

B. an itchy, swollen lesion that lasts only a few hours

C. an open lesion on the skin accompanied by loss of skin depth

D. a small, elevated pimple in the skin

E. a crack in the skin such as in chapped hands or lips

F. the scab on a sore

G. likely to form after the healing of an injury

H. an elevation of the skin having an inflamed base, containing pus

I. an external swelling, varying in size, shape, and color

J. a small, discolored spot or patch such as freckles

K. a blister similar to but larger than a vesicle

L. a blister with clear fluid in it

Word Review: The student is encouraged to write down the meaning of each of the following words. The list can be used as a study guide for this unit.

collagen	keratin	stratum germinativum
cuticle	malpighian	stratum granulosum
dermis	melanin	subcutaneous tissue
epidermis	reticular layer	sudoriferous
integument	sebaceous	

System Two: The Skeletal System

Short Answer: List the five main functions of the skeletal system.

1. _____

2. _____

3. _____

   _____

4. _____

5. _____

Key Choices: Classify each of the following bones in one of four major bone categories by placing the appropriate letter in the space provided.

S = Short bones   I = Irregular bones
L = Long bones   F = Flat bones

_____ 1. tibia   _____ 7. axis

_____ 2. ilium   _____ 8. femur

_____ 3. phalange   _____ 9. talus

_____ 4. ulna   _____ 10. metacarpal

_____ 5. occiput   _____ 11. scapula

_____ 6. calcaneus   _____ 12. rib

Completion: In the space provided, write the word or words that correctly complete each statement.

1. The skeletal system is composed of _____ and _____.

2. The inorganic mineral matter of bone consists mainly of _____ and _____.

3. The fibrous membrane covering bone that serves as an attachment for tendons and ligaments is the _____.

4. The spongy bone tissue in flat bones and at the ends of long bones is filled with _____ and is the sight of production for _____.

5. The hollow chamber formed in the shaft of long bones that is filled with yellow bone marrow is the _____.

Identification: Figure 5.6 is a diagram of a typical long bone. Identify the indicated structures and write the correct letters in the space provided.

_____ 1. proximal epiphysis

_____ 2. compact bone

_____ 3. diaphysis (shaft of bone)

_____ 4. epiphyseal plate (site of longitudinal bone growth in children)

_____ 5. distal epiphysis

_____ 6. medullary cavity (site of yellow bone marrow in adults)

_____ 7. periosteum (covering of bone)

_____ 8. spongy bone (site of red bone marrow)

_____ 9. nutrient

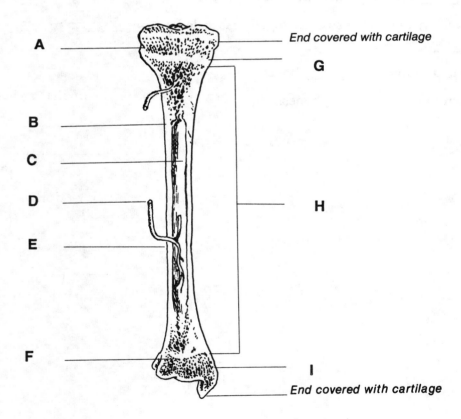

Fig. 5.6   Structure of long bone.

Completion: In the space provided, write the word or words that correctly complete each statement.

1. The two main parts of the skeleton are the _____ and the _____ _____.

2. The bones of the skull, thorax, vertebral column, and the hyoid bone comprise the _____ _____.

3. The bones of the shoulder, upper extremities, hips, and lower extremities make up the _____.

4. In the human adult, the skeleton consists of _____ bones.

5. The spine consists of _____ vertebra.

6. There are _____ cervical vertebra.

7. There are _____ thoracic vertebra.

8. There are _____ lumbar vertebra.

9. There are _____ carpals in each wrist.

10. There are _____ tarsals in each ankle.

11. There are _____ phalanges in each hand.

12. The connection where two bones come together is called a _____ or an _____.

13. The cranium is composed of _____ bones.

14. The face is composed of _____ bones.

Key Choices: Joints are classified according to the amount of motion they permit. In the space provided, place the appropriate letter next to the corresponding term(s).

A = Amphiarthrotic joints

D = Diarthrotic joints

S = Synarthrotic joints

_____ 1. symphysis pubis

_____ 2. glenohumeral joint

_____ 3. sagittal suture

_____ 4. elbow joint

_____ 5. bones united by fibrous connective tissue

_____ 6. hip joint

_____ 7. essentially immovable

_____ 8. sacroiliac joint

_____ 9. joint capsule with synovial fluid

_____ 10. intervertebral joints

_____ 11. articular cartilage on bones

_____ 12. joint between sphenoid and temporal bones

_____ 13. freely movable

_____ 14. allows limited movement

Key Choice: In the space provided, write the letter that corresponds to the appropriate classification of joint. Movable joints in the body are classified as:

A. pivot joints   C. hinge joints   E. saddle joints

B. ball and socket joints   D. gliding joints

_____ 1. joint between ulna and humerus

_____ 2. hip joint

_____ 3. knee joint

_____ 4. joint between the first metacarpal and the trapezium

_____ 5. joints between radius and carpals

_____ 6. glenohumeral joint

_____ 7. joint between axis and atlas

_____ 8. joint between radius and ulna near elbow

_____ 9. intervertebral joints

_____ 10. interphalangeal joints

_____ 11. joint between the tibia and the talus

Identification: Identify the bones in Figure 5.7 by writing the correct label in the numbered space that corresponds to the number on the diagram.

1. _____	11. _____	21. _____
2. _____	12. _____	22. _____
3. _____	13. _____	23. _____
4. _____	14. _____	24. _____
5. _____	15. _____	25. _____
6. _____	16. _____	26. _____
7. _____	17. _____	27. _____
8. _____	18. _____	28. _____
9. _____	19. _____	29. _____
10. _____	20. _____	

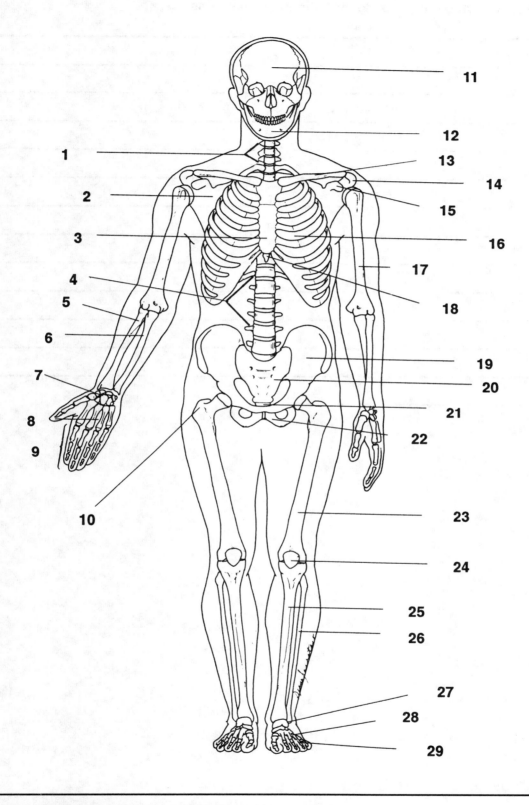

Fig. 5.7   Skeletal system, anterior view.

Identification: Identify the bony landmarks in Figures 5.8a and 5.8b by writing the correct name in the lettered space that corresponds to the letter in the diagrams.

A. _____   N. _____

B. _____   O. _____

C. _____   P. _____

D. _____   Q. _____

_____   R. _____

E. _____   S. _____

F. _____   T. _____

G. _____   U. _____

H. _____   V. _____

I. _____   W. _____

J. _____   X. _____

K. _____   Y. _____

L. _____   Z. _____

M. _____

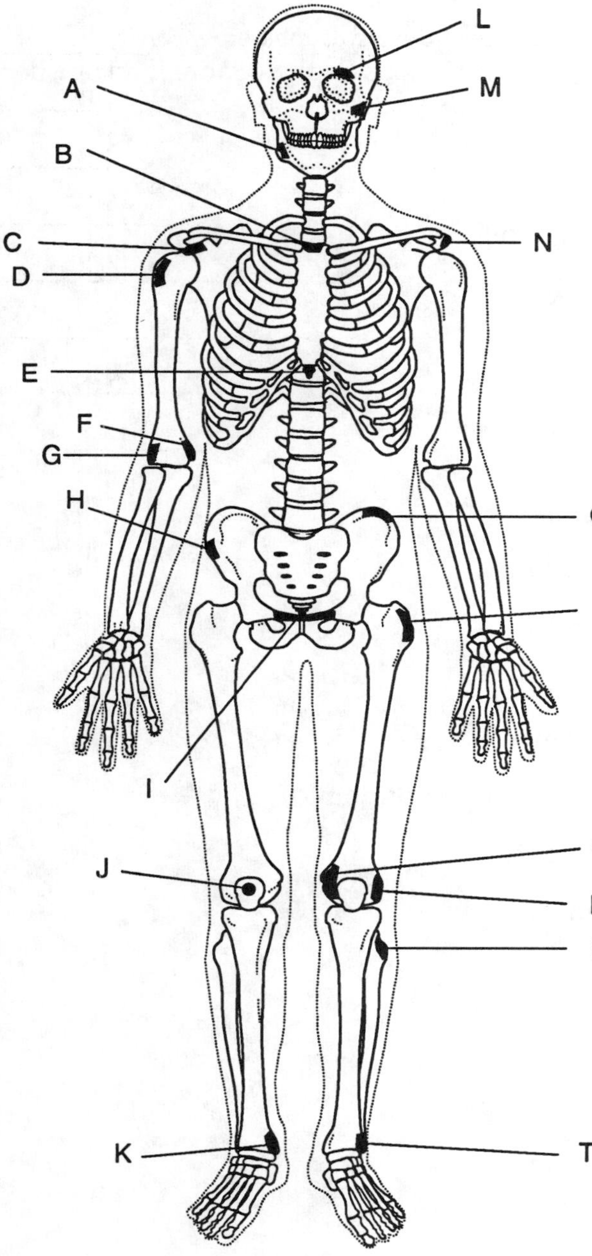

Fig. 5.8a Major bony landmarks on the body, anterior view.

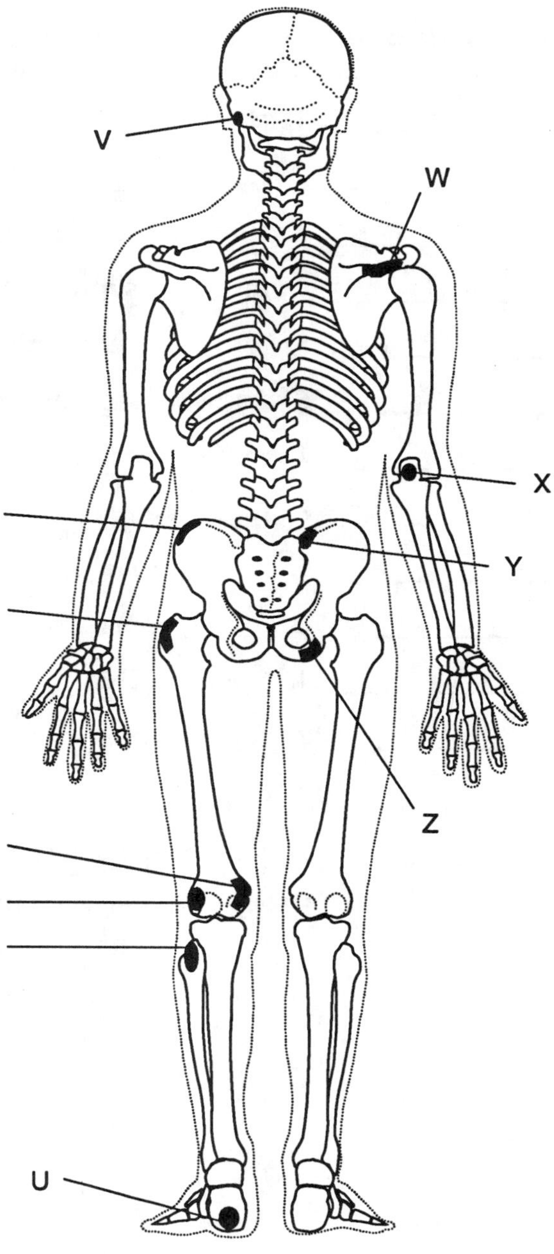

Fig. 5.8b Major bony landmarks on the body, posterior view.

Identification: Identify the bones in Figure 5.9 by writing the correct number next to the appropriate name.

_____ A. ethmoid

_____ B. frontal

_____ C. hyoid

_____ D. vertebral section

_____ E. lacrimal

_____ F. mandible

_____ G. maxilla

_____ H. nasal

_____ I. occipital

_____ J. parietal

_____ K. sphenoid

_____ L. temporal

_____ M. zygomatic

Matching: Match the bone names listed above with the best descriptions below. Write the letter of the bone name in the space provided. Note that some descriptions apply to more than one bone.

_____ 1. cheek bone

_____ 2. holds the upper teeth

_____ 3. contains the foramen magnum

_____ 4. forms the supraorbital ridge

_____ 5. four bones containing sinuses

_____ 6. forms the sagittal suture

_____ 7. forms the coronal suture

_____ 8. forms the squamosal suture

_____ 9. forms the lambdoidal suture

_____ 10. forms the mastoid process

_____ 11. forms the chin

_____ 12. connects with all other cranial bones

_____ 13. connected to the skull with a diarthrotic joint

_____ 14. contain openings for tear ducts

_____ 15. does not connect with any other bone

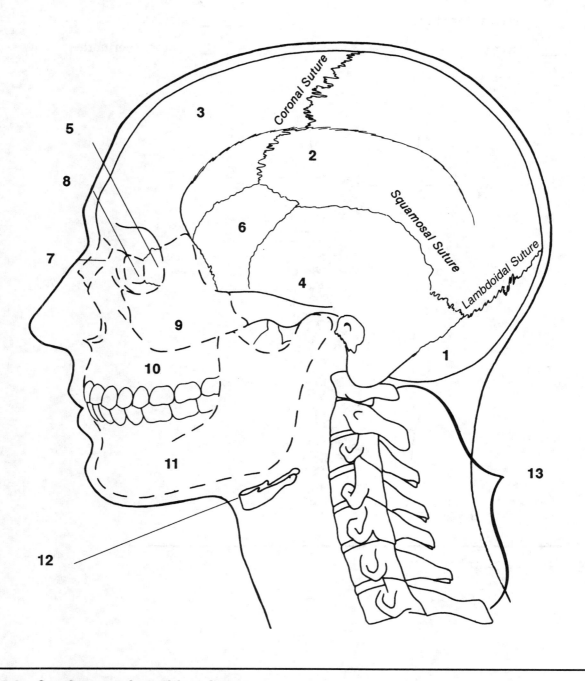

Fig. 5.9   Cranium, neck, and face bones.

Identification: Identify the parts of the spine in Figure 5.10 by writing the correct letter next to the corresponding label in the space provided.

_____ atlas axis   _____ lumbar vertebrae

_____ cervical vertebrae   _____ sacrum

_____ coccyx   _____ thoracic vertebrae

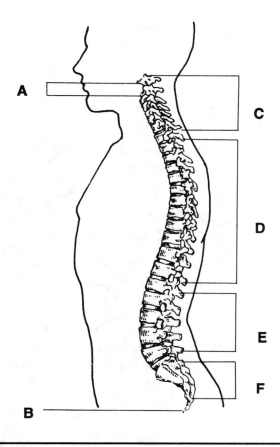

Fig. 5.10 Vertebral column.

Matching: Match the term with the best description. Write the letter of the best description in the space provided.

_____ 1. fossa

_____ 2. trochanter

_____ 3. foramen

_____ 4. sinus

_____ 5. process

_____ 6. condyle

_____ 7. line

_____ 8. tuberosity

_____ 9. meatus

_____ 10. tubercle

_____ 11. head

_____ 12. spine

_____ 13. crest

A. a less prominent ridge of a bone than a crest

B. a rounded articulating process at the end of a bone

C. a large process for muscle attachment

D. a sharp slender projection

E. a tubelike passage

F. a depression or hollow

G. a ridge

H. a cavity within a bone

I. a rounded knuckle-like prominence usually at a point of articulation

J. a small rounded process

K. a hole

L. a large rounded process

M. a bone prominence or projection

Short Answer: Circle the term that does not belong in each of the following groupings.

tibia	patella	femur	fibula
elbow	knee	finger	hip
axis/atlas	sacroiliac	intervertebral	pubic symphysis
tubercle	fossa	tuberosity	condyle
cranium	rib	vertebra	scapula

Key Choices: Identify the skeletal disorders by writing the appropriate letter in the space provided.

A. dislocation   C. osteoarthritis   E. fractures   G. bursitis

B. sprain   D. osteoporosis   F. rheumatoid arthritis

_____ 1. an inflammation of the small fluid-filled sacs located near the joints

_____ 2. a break or rupture in a bone

_____ 3. an inflammation causing the articular cartilage to erode and the joints to calcify and eventually become immovable

_____ 4. increased porosity of the bone that causes a thinning of bone tissue

_____ 5. displacement of a bone within a joint

_____ 6. a chronic inflammatory disease, that first affects the synovial membrane lining the joints

_____ 7. stretching or tearing of ligaments

_____ 8. a chronic disease that accompanies aging, usually affecting joints that have experienced a great deal of wear and tear or trauma

Identification: Identify each of the spinal curves in Figure 5.11 by writing the correct label in the space provided.

A. _____ B. _____ C. _____

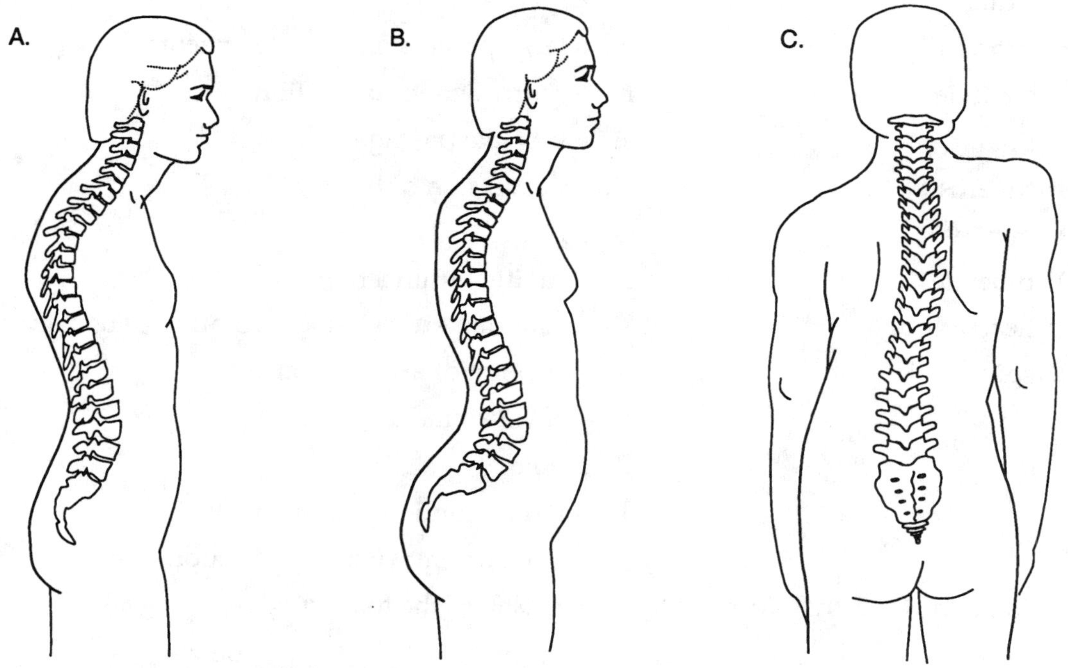

Fig. 5.11 Abnormal curvatures of the spine.

Word Review: The student is encouraged to write down the meaning of each of the following words. The list can be used as a study guide for this unit.

ampiarthrotic	cranium	medullary cavity
appendicular skeleton	diaphysis	periosteum
arthritis	diarthrotic	osteoporosis
articular cartilage	epiphysis	scoliosis
articulation	joint capsule	sprain
axial skeleton	kyphosis	synarthrotic
bursa	ligament	synovial fluid
cartilage	lordosis	synovial membrane
compact bone tissue	marrow	vertebra

System Three: The Muscular System

Key Choices: Identify the muscle type described by writing the correct letter(s) in the space provided.

A. skeletal   B. smooth   C. cardiac

_____ 1. contains striations

_____ 2. shapes and contours the body

_____ 3. forms the hollow organs

_____ 4. involved with transport of materials in the body

_____ 5. found only in the heart

_____ 6. spindle shaped

_____ 7. multinucleated

_____ 8. controlled by the autonomic nervous system

_____ 9. quadrangular in shape, joined end to end

_____ 10. contracts without direct nerve action

_____ 11. referred to as the muscular system

_____ 12. coordinates activity to act as a pump

Completion: In the space provided, write the word or words that correctly complete each statement.

1. The main organ of the muscle system is _____.

2. Muscle cells have the unique ability to _____.

3. Muscle comprises approximately _____ percent of a person's body weight.

4. The characteristics that enable muscles to perform their functions of contraction and movement are _____,_____ and _____.

5. The ability to return to its original shape after being stretched is _____.

6. The capacity of muscles to receive and react to stimuli is _____.

7. The ability to contract or shorten and thereby exert force is _____.

Structure of Skeletal Muscles

Identification: Identify each skeletal muscle part in Figure 5.12 by writing the appropriate number next to the correct term in the space provided.

_____ A. endomysium   _____ E. myofibril   _____ I. sarcoplasm

_____ B. epimysium   _____ F. muscle fiber   _____ J. tendon

_____ C. fascicle   _____ G. perimysium

_____ D. myofilament   _____ H. sarcolemma

Matching: Using the terms listed above, write the letter of the appropriate term in the space provided.

_____ 1. connective tissue projecting beyond the end of the muscle

_____ 2. connective tissue covering the entire muscle

_____ 3. separates muscles into bundles of fibers

_____ 4. connective tissue covering of each muscle cell

_____ 5. bundle of muscle fibers

_____ 6. contractile unit of muscle tissue

_____ 7. one of the microscopic threads that can be rendered visible in a muscle fiber

_____ 8. the muscle cell membrane

_____ 9. structure of the muscle cell containing actin and myosin

_____ 10. the muscle cell intercellular fluid

Completion: In the space provided, write the word or words that correctly complete each statement.

1. The functional unit of a muscle is the _____ or _____.

2. The cell membrane of the muscle cell is the _____.

3. The connective tissue covering of the muscle cell is the _____.

4. Each muscle cell contains hundreds or even thousands of parallel _____.

5. The interaction of _____ and _____ filaments gives muscle its unique contractile ability.

6. The arrangement of _____ and _____ gives skeletal muscles a striated or striped appearance.

7. The site where the muscle fiber and nerve fiber meet is called the _____ or _____.

8. A motor neuron and all the muscle fibers that it controls constitute a _____.

9. When a nerve impulse reaches the end of the nerve fiber, a chemical neurotransmitter called _____ is released.

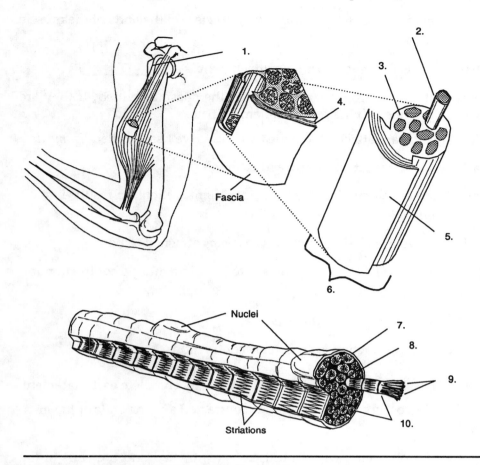

Fig. 5.12   Structure of skeletal muscle.

10. The energy for muscle contraction comes from the breakdown of the _____
    _____ .

11. A metabolic process known as the _____ or the _____ takes place
    resulting in the synthesis of ATP, and the production of carbon dioxide, water, and energy in
    the form of heat.

12. When sufficient oxygen is available, ATP is synthesized through _____ respiration.

13. When the oxygen supply is depleted, ATP is synthesized through _____
    respiration.

14. During strenuous activity heavy breathing and accelerated heart rate are indications of
    _____ .

15. Rapid or prolonged muscle contractions, to the point that oxygen debt becomes extreme and
    the muscle ceases to respond, causes _____ .

16. A muscle that is firm and responds promptly to stimulation under normal conditions has
    good _____ .

17. The most stationary attachment of a muscle is the _____ .

18. The muscle attachment that creates the action of the structure is the _____ .

19. A(n) _____ contraction occurs when a muscle contracts and the ends of the muscle do not move.

20. The glistening cord that connects the muscle with its attachment is a _____.

True or False: If the following statements are true, write *true* in the space provided. If they are false, replace the italicized word with one that makes the statement true.

_____ 1. Muscle fibers are attached to bone by connective tissue called *ligaments*.

_____ 2. Each motor nerve attaches to *one* muscle cell.

_____ 3. The release of calcium ions by the sarcoplasmic reticulum results in a *muscle contraction*.

_____ 4. A skeletal muscle by definition has *both ends* attached to bone.

_____ 5. Only enough ATP is stored in muscle to sustain a muscle contraction for a few *minutes*.

_____ 6. ATP is produced by the *mitochondria*.

_____ 7. An eccentric contraction is an *isotonic* contraction.

Completion: In the space provided, write the word or words that correctly complete each statement.

1. A(n) _____ contraction occurs when a muscle is contracted and the ends of the muscle move further apart.

2. A(n) _____ contraction occurs when a muscle is contracted and the ends of the muscle move closer together.

3. Eccentric and concentric muscle contractions are both _____ contractions.

4. When an action occurs, the muscle that is responsible for that action is the _____ _____.

5. When an action occurs, the muscle that is responsible for the opposite action is the _____.

6. Muscles that assist the primary muscle of an action are called _____.

7. When discussing the dynamics of the movement of the body, the three components of motion are _____ and _____.

Matching: Match the term with the best description. Write the letter of the best description in the space provided.

_____ 1. posterior	A. that which presses or draws down
_____ 2. dilator	B. behind or in back of
_____ 3. inferior	C. pertaining to the middle or center
_____ 4. anguli	D. before or in front of
_____ 5. levator	E. situated lower
_____ 6. dorsal	F. to straighten
_____ 7. superior	G. that which lifts
_____ 8. medial	H. behind or in back of
_____ 9. distal	I. nearer to the center or medial line
_____ 10. depressor	J. at an angle
_____ 11. proximal	K. farther from the center or medial line
_____ 12. anterior	L. situated above
_____ 13. extensor	M. that which expands or enlarges

Matching: Match the term with the best description. Write the letter of the appropriate term in the space provided.

A. flexion	E. adduction	I. medial rotation	M. inversion
B. extension	F. abduction	J. lateral rotation	N. eversion
C. dorsi flexion	G. pronation	K. circumduction	O. elevation
D. plantar flexion	H. supination	L. hyperextension	P. depression

_____ 1. raise the shoulders toward the ears

_____ 2. action of the neck when looking at the ceiling

_____ 3. action of the hip when standing up out of a seated position

_____ 4. action of the toes when standing on tiptoes

_____ 5. turning the hand palm up

_____ 6. action of the foot when pointing toes

_____ 7. action of elbow during eccentric contraction of bicep

_____ 8. bringing the knees together

_____ 9. action of knee during concentric contraction of biceps femoris

_____ 10. turning the sole of the foot medially

_____ 11. action of the femur when turning the feet outward

_____ 12. action of the hip when bringing the knee toward the chest

_____ 13. turning the palm of the hand downward

_____ 14. action of the foot when pointing the toes up toward the knee

Identification: Identify the muscles in Figure 5.13 by writing the correct name in the space provided.

The Muscular System—Anterior View

1. _____   15. _____

2. _____   16. _____

3. _____   17. _____

4. _____   18. _____

5. _____   19. _____

6. _____   20. _____

7. _____   21. _____

8. _____   22. _____

9. _____   23. _____

10. _____   24. _____

11. _____   25. _____

12. _____   26. _____

13. _____   27. _____

14. _____

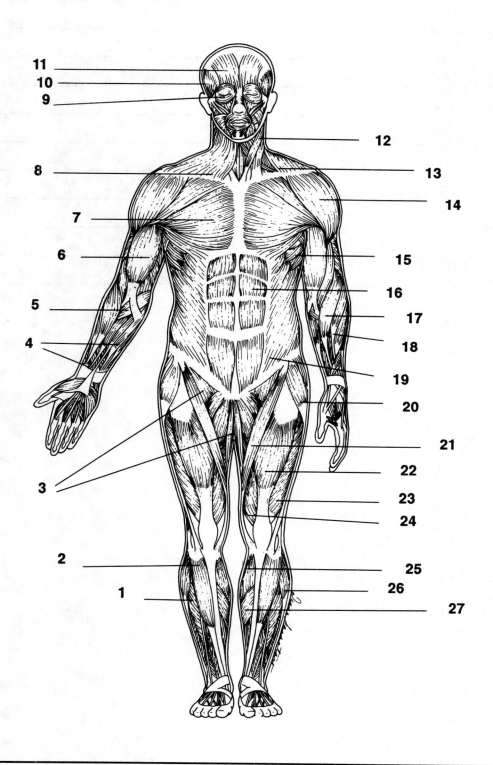

Fig. 5.13   The muscular system, anterior view.

Identification: Identify the muscles in Figure 5.14 by writing the correct name in the space provided.

The Muscular System—Posterior View

1. _____   12. _____

2. _____   13. _____

3. _____   14. _____

4. _____   15. _____

5. _____   16. _____

6. _____   17. _____

7. _____   18. _____

8. _____   19. _____

9. _____   20. _____

10. _____   21. _____

11. _____   22. _____

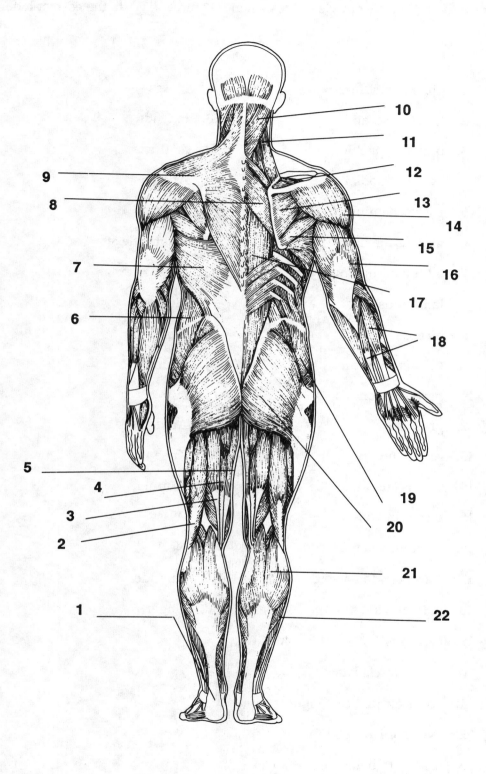

Fig. 5.14   The muscular system, posterior view.

Matching: In the first answer column, identify the body part the muscle acts on. In the second answer column indicate the action the muscle causes when it contracts. Write the correct letter in the answer blank.

Body part   Action

_____ _____   1. gluteus medius   A. Flexes

_____ _____   2. triceps brachii   B. Extends

_____ _____   3. upper trapezius   C. Adducts

_____ _____   4. deltoid (medial)   D. Abducts

_____ _____   5. gastrocnemius   E. Elevates

_____ _____   6. gluteus maximus   F. Plantar flexes

_____ _____   7. adductor magnus   G. Dorsal flexes

_____ _____   8. latissimus dorsi   H. Big toe

_____ _____   9. biceps femoris   I. Elbow

_____ _____   10. tibialis anterior   J. Thumb

_____ _____   11. peroneus longus   K. Hip

_____ _____   12. gracilis   L. Ankle

_____ _____   13. rectus femoris   M. Knee

_____ _____   14. vastus lateralis   N. Scapula

_____ _____   15. biceps brachii   O. Wrist

_____ _____   16. pectoralis major   P. Neck

_____ _____   17. sternocleidomastoid   Q. Shoulder

_____ _____   18. palmaris longus   R. Finger

_____ _____   19. sartorius

_____ _____   20. tensor fascia lata

_____ _____   21. abductor pollicis longus

_____ _____   22. extensor hallucis longus

_____ _____   23. brachioradialis

_____ _____   24. extensor indicus

_____ _____   25. soleus

_____ _____   26. iliopsoas

_____ _____   27. supraspinatus

Completion: In the space provided, write the word or words that correctly complete each statement.

1.   A sudden involuntary contraction of a muscle or a group of muscles is a _____.

2.   An enlargement of the breadth of a muscle as a result of repeated forceful muscle activity is called _____.

3.   When the muscle tissue degenerates and begins to waste away, the process is called _____.

4.   The process where muscle tissue is replaced by fibrous connective tissue is _____.

5.   Two inflammatory conditions of the white fibrous tissue which cause pain and stiffness, [especially the fascial tissues of the muscular system], are _____ and _____.

6.   A group of related diseases that seem to be genetically inherited and that cause a progressive degeneration of the voluntary muscular system is _____.

Short Answer: Circle the term that does not belong in each of the following groups.

brachioradialis	biceps brachii	brachialis	coracobrachialis
biceps femoris	rectus femoris	vastus medialis	vastus lateralis
supraspinatus	subscapularis	teres major	teres minor
pectineus	rectus femoris	adductor longus	gracilis
teres major	pectoralis major	subscapularis	infraspinatus

Identification: On the skeleton diagrams in Figures 5.15a through 5.16b, draw by shading the indicated muscles. Be as accurate as possible, paying close attention to muscle attachments. Draw the muscles on the indicated sides to minimize overlap.

Note that the right hand of all of the diagrams are supinated.

Right Hand Side	Left Hand Side
A. tibialis anterior	J. pectoralis minor
B. gracilis	K. coracobrachialis
C. adductor longus	L. rectus abdominis
D. pectineus	M. flexor digitorum profundus
E. tensor fascia latae	N. adductor brevis
F. flexor carpi ulnaris	O. adductor magnus
G. external obliques	P. extensor digitorum longus
H. biceps brachii	
I. serratus anterior	

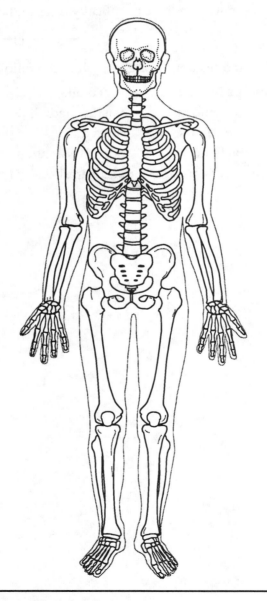

Fig. 5.15a   The skeletal system, anterior view.

Right Hand Side

A. peroneus brevis
B. extensor hallucis longus
C. vastus lateralis
D. vastus medialis
E. flexor digitorum superficialis
F. iliacus
G. psoas
H. pectoralis major
I. sternocleidomastoid

Left Hand Side

J. deltoid
K. brachialis
L. quadratus lumborum
M. flexor carpi radialis
N. rectus femoris
O. peroneus longus

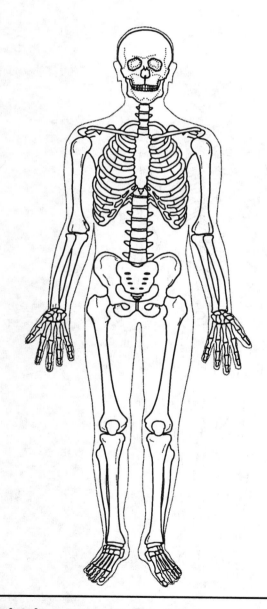

Fig. 5.15b   The skeletal system, anterior view.

Left Hand Side

A. flexor digitorum longus

B. biceps femoris

C. emimembranosis

D. gluteus medius

E. brachioradialis

F. latissimus dorsi

G. rhomboids

H. levator scapulae

Right Hand Side

I. trapezius

J. teres major

K. extensor carpi radialis brevis

L. extensor carpi ulnaris

M. gluteus minimus

N. piriformis

O. semitendinosis

P. popliteus

Q. posterior tibialis

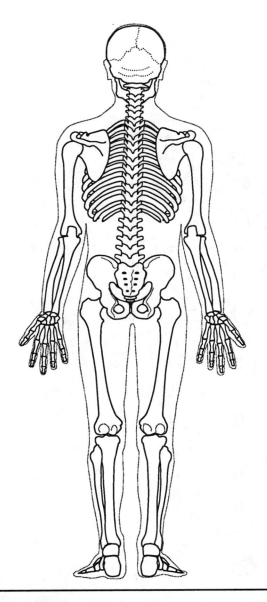

Fig. 5.16a   The skeletal system, posterior view.

Left Hand Side

A. gastrocnemius

B. quadratus femoris

C. extensor carpi radialis longus

D. triceps

E. infraspinatus

F. supraspinatus

G. erector spini

Right Hand Side

H. spleneus capitis

I. teres minor

J. extensor digitorum

K. gluteus maximus

L. iliotibial band

M. soleus

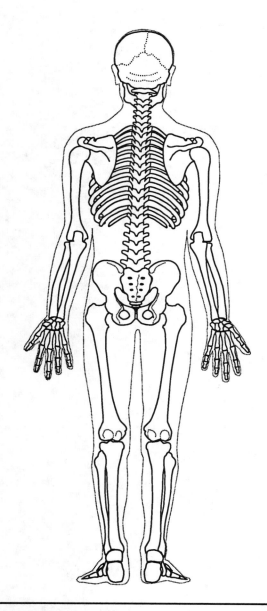

Fig. 5.16b   The skeletal system, posterior view.

Word Review: The student is encouraged to write down the meaning of each of the following words. The list can be used as a study guide for this unit.

abduction	fascia	origin
adduction	flexion	oxygen debt
actin	insertion	prime mover
antagonist	motor neuron	pronation
aponeurosis	motor unit	skeletal muscle
cardiac muscle	muscle belly	smooth muscle
contractility	muscle fatigue	striated
elasticity	muscle tone	supination
extensibility	myofibril	synergist
extension	myosin	tendon

System Four: The Circulatory System

Completion: In the space provided, write the word or words that correctly complete each statement.

1. The two divisions to the vascular system are the _____

    _____ and _____ .

2. The double-layered membrane that covers the heart is the _____ .

3. The normal heart rate for an adult is _____ beats per minute.

4. The blood vessels that carry blood away from the heart are _____ and _____ .

5. The blood vessels that carry blood back toward the heart are _____ and _____ .

6. The largest artery in the body is the _____ .

7. The smallest, microscopic, thin-walled blood vessels are called _____ .

8. The two circulation systems in the blood vascular system are _____

    and _____ .

Identification: Figure 5.17 shows a cross section of a portion of the heart wall including the pericardium. Identify the following parts indicated on the diagram by writing the appropriate letter in the space provided.

_____ 1. epicardium   _____ 4. parietal pericardium

_____ 2. myocardium   _____ 5. pericardial cavity

_____ 3. endocardium   _____ 6. visceral pericardium

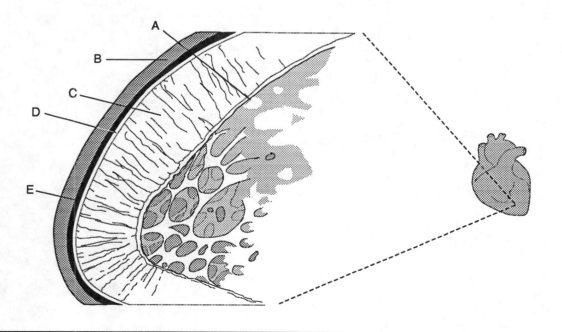

Fig. 5.17   Cross-section of wall of heart.

Identification: Figure 5.18 is a diagram of a frontal section of the heart. Identify each indicated structure of the heart by writing the correct letter next to the corresponding term.

_____	1. aorta	_____	9. pulmonary semilunar valve
_____	2. aortic semilunar valve	_____	10. pulmonary vein
_____	3. bicuspid valve	_____	11. right atrium
_____	4. inferior vena cava	_____	12. right ventricle
_____	5. left atrium	_____	13. septum
_____	6. left ventricle	_____	14. superior vena cava
_____	7. mitral valve	_____	15. tricuspid valve
_____	8. pulmonary artery		

Identification: On Figure 5.18 draw arrows to indicate the direction in which blood flows through the heart. Use dotted arrows for oxygen-rich blood and solid arrows for oxygen-poor blood.

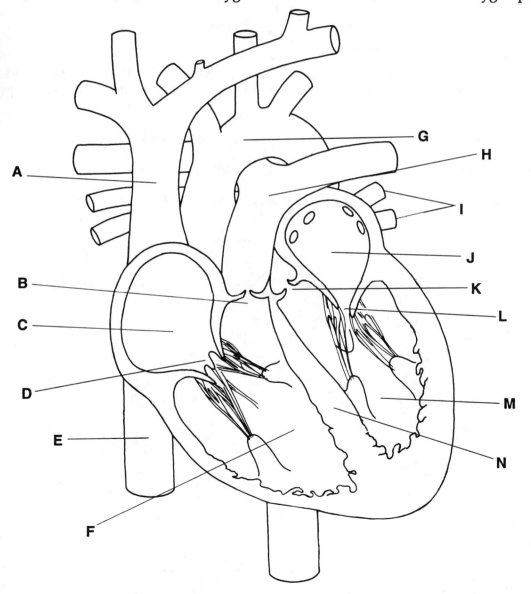

Fig. 5.18   Frontal section of the heart.

True or False: If the following statements are true, write *true* in the space provided. If they are false, replace the italicized word with one that makes the statement true.

_____ 1. Impulses from the sympathetic portion of the autonomic nervous system cause *vasodilatation* and increased blood flow.

_____ 2. Substances move through the capillary walls mostly by *osmosis*.

_____ 3. Blood moves through the *arterioles* to the capillaries and then to the *venules*.

_____ 4. *Diffusion* is a process where substances move from an area of higher pressure to lower pressure.

_____ 5. In *pulmonary* circulation, veins contain oxygen-rich blood.

Matching: Match the term with the best description. Write the letter of the appropriate term in the space provided.

A. arteriosclerosis   C. embolus   E. atherosclerosis
B. phlebitis   D. varicose veins   F. edema

_____ 1. protruding, bulbous, distended superficial veins

_____ 2. an inflammation of a vein

_____ 3. a condition of excess fluid in the interstitial spaces

_____ 4. the walls of affected arteries tend to thicken, become fibrous and loose their elasticity

_____ 5. an accumulation of fatty deposits on the inner walls of the arteries

_____ 6. clots that break loose and float in the blood

True or False: If the following statements are true, write *true* in the space provided. If they are false, replace the italicized word with one that makes the statement true.

_____ 1. The cardio-vascular system of the average adult male contains about *four* liters of blood.

_____ 2. Blood has a slightly *acid* reaction.

_____ 3. Plasma accounts for *75* percent of the blood's volume.

_____ 4. *White blood cells* make up as much as 95 percent of all blood cells.

_____ 5. Red blood cells and *white blood cells* are produced in the red bone marrow.

Short Answer: Five functions of the blood are listed below. In the space provided, briefly describe how the blood performs these functions.

1. Blood provides nutrients to the cells.

   _____

2. Blood removes wastes.

   _____

   _____

3. Blood maintains normal body temperature.

_____

_____

4. Blood protects against infection.

_____

5. Blood prevents hemorrhaging.

_____

Completion: In the space provided, write the word or words that correctly complete each statement.

1. The red blood cells are also called _____.

2. Red blood cells are colored with an oxygen-carrying substance called _____.

3. The process where leukocytes actually engulf and digest harmful bacteria is called _____.

4. The small irregularly shaped particles in the blood that play an important role in clotting are _____ or _____.

5. A disease characterized by extremely slow clotting of blood and excessive bleeding from even very slight cuts is _____.

6. A condition in which there is a rapid loss or inadequate production of red blood cells is _____.

7. A form of cancer in which there is an uncontrolled production of white blood cells is known as _____.

Identification: Figure 5.19 is a diagram of the major blood vessels of the body. The arteries are indicated on the left side of the body as unshaded vessels. The veins are indicated on the right side of the body as shaded vessels. Identify the numbered blood vessels and write the correct name on the line next to the identifying number.

1. _____   12. _____
2. _____   13. _____
3. _____   14. _____
4. _____   15. _____
5. _____   16. _____
6. _____   17. _____
7. _____   18. _____
8. _____   19. _____
9. _____   20. _____
10. _____   21. _____
11. _____

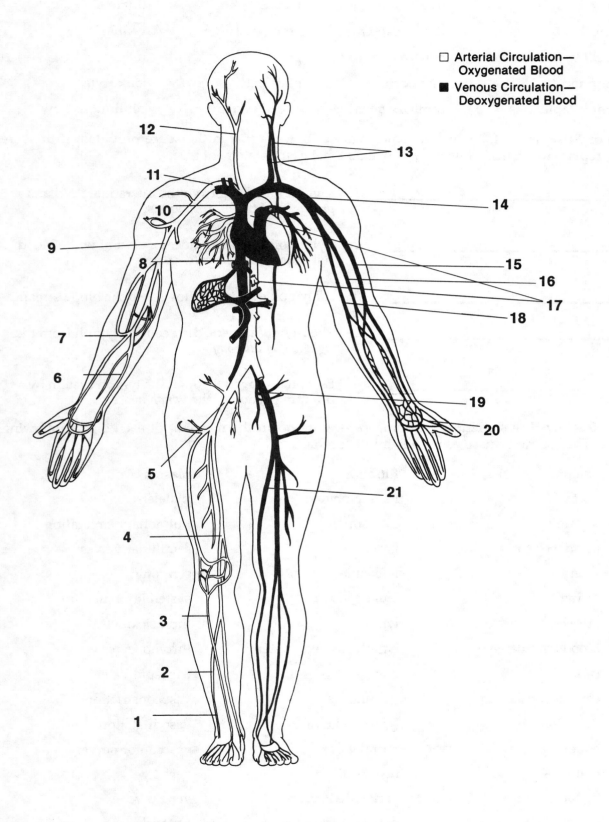

□ Arterial Circulation—
Oxygenated Blood
■ Venous Circulation—
Deoxygenated Blood

Fig. 5.19 Circulatory system.

Short Answer: Circle the term that does not belong in the following word groups.

spleen	liver	tonsils	thymus
lacteal	thoracic duct	lymphatic	venule
swelling	nausea	pain	redness
lymphocytes	monocytes	platelets	leukocytes
lymph capillaries	capillary beds	closed system	continuous flow

True or False: If the following statements are true, write *true* in the space provided. If they are false, replace the italicized word with one that makes the statement true.

_____ 1. Lymph is derived from the interstitial fluid and *produced* by the lymph nodes.

_____ 2. Lymphoid tissue produces a kind of white blood cell called a *lymphocyte.*

_____ 3. *All* lymph eventually flows into the blood stream.

_____ 4. The right lymphatic duct collects lymph from the *right half of the body*.

_____ 5. Lymph is moved through the lymph system by a pumping action of the *lymph nodes.*

Word Review: The student is encouraged to write down the meaning of each of the following words. The list can be used as a study guide for this unit.

anemia	filtration	plasma
aorta	hemoglobin	platelets
arteriole	interstitial	pulmonary circulation
arteriosclerosis	lacteal	semilunar valves
artery	leukemia	seratonin
atrium	leukocytes	systemic circulation
auricle	lymph	thoracic duct
blood vascular system	lymph vascular system	thrombocytes
capillary	lymphatic pump	tricuspid valve
cardiovascular	lymphatics	vasoconstriction
diffusion	lymphoid tissue	vasodilatation
edema	mitral valve	vasomotor nerves
embolus	myocardium	vein
endocardium	pericardial cavity	vena cava
epicardium	pericardium	ventricle
erythrocytes	phagocytosis	venule
fibrin	phlebitis	

System Five: The Nervous System

Completion: In the space provided, write the word or words that correctly complete each statement.

1. The major parts of the nervous system are the _____ and _____.

2. The structural unit of the nervous system is the _____ or _____.

3. There are two types of nerve fibers. _____ connect with other neurons to receive information and a single _____ conducts impulses away from the cell body.

4. Impulses are passed from one neuron to another at a junction called a _____.

5. Two characteristics of a neuron are _____ and _____.

6. Neurons that originate in the periphery and carry information toward the central nervous system [CNS] are _____ or _____ neurons.

7. Neurons that carry impulses from the brain to the muscles or glands that they control are _____ or _____ neurons.

8. Neurons located in the brain and spinal cord that carry impulses from one neuron to another are _____ or _____ neurons.

9. The portion of the nervous system that is surrounded by bone is the _____ which consists of the _____ and the _____.

10. The CNS is covered by a special connective tissue membrane called the _____, which has three layers: the _____, the _____, and the _____.

11. The fluid that surrounds and supports the brain and spinal cord is _____.

12. The largest portion making up the front and top of the brain is the _____.

13. The smaller part of the brain that helps maintain body balance and coordinates voluntary muscles is the _____.

14. The three parts of the brain stem are the _____, the _____, and the _____.

15. The two divisions of the peripheral nervous system are the _____, which involves the nerves to the visceral organs, glands, and blood vessels, and the _____, which involves the nerves to the muscles and skin.

Identification: Figure 5.20 is a diagram of a nerve cell. Identify the indicated structures by writing the letter of the structures next to the correct term.

_____ 1. axon

_____ 2. axon branches

_____ 3. cell body

_____ 4. dendrites

_____ 5. protective fatty sheath

_____ 6. nucleus

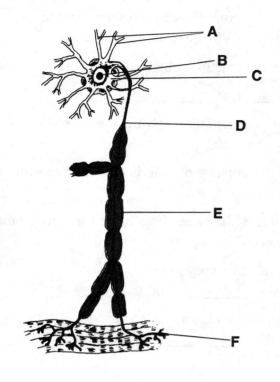

Fig. 5.20   Nerve cell.

Matching: Match the term with the best description. Write the letter of the appropriate term in the space provided.

A. afferent neuron   D. efferent neuron   G. nerve

B. axon   E. ganglion   H. stimuli

C. dendrite   F. interneuron   I. synapse

_____ 1. the conducting portion of a neuron

_____ 2. junction point between neurons

_____ 3. bundle of axons in the peripheral nervous system

_____ 4. collection of nerve bodies located outside of the CNS

_____ 5. changes that activate the nervous system

_____ 6. receptive structure of the neuron

_____ 7. carries sensory information toward the CNS

_____ 8. transmits information from one neuron to another

True or False: If the following statements are true, write *true* in the space provided. If they are false, replace the italicized word with one that makes the statement true.

_____ 1. The spinal cord extends from the medulla oblongata to the *sacrum*.

_____ 2. Control centers in the *pons* regulate movements of the heart and control vasoconstriction of the arteries.

_____ 3. The *midbrain* relays impulses from the cerebrum to the cerebellum.

_____ 4. Spinal nerves are numbered according to *the level where they exit the spine*.

_____ 5. There are *thirty-one* pairs of spinal nerves.

_____ 6. All of the nerves outside of the brain and spinal cord are considered to be the *peripheral* nervous system.

Cranial Nerves

Identification and Matching: Number the cranial nerves according to the order in which they arise from the brain. In the first column of answer blanks, write the Roman numeral that corresponds to the cranial nerve. Then, select the best description of the function of the cranial nerve and write the appropriate letter in the second column of answer blanks.

Number Function

_____ _____ 1. trochlear nerve

_____ _____ 2. optic nerve

_____ _____ 3. hypoglossal nerve

_____ _____ 4. vagus nerve

_____ _____ 5. accessory nerve

_____ _____ 6. abducens nerve

_____ _____ 7. oculomotor nerve

_____ _____ 8. trigeminal nerve

_____ _____ 9. auditory nerve

_____ _____ 10. olfactory nerve

_____ _____ 11. glossopharyngeal nerve

_____ _____ 12. facial nerve

A. speaking, shoulder, and neck muscles

B. sensations of the face and movement of the jaw and tongue

C. moves eyeball up and out

D. sensation and movement related to talking, heart rate, breathing and digestion

E. sense of smell

F. moves eyeball up, down and in, constricts pupil, raises eyelid

G. tongue movement, and swallowing

H. movements of the face, and salivary glands

I. moves eyeball outward

J. tongue movement, swallowing, sense of taste

K. sense of sight

L. sense of hearing

Short Answer: Write the answers to the following questions in the space provided.

1. How many pairs of cervical nerves are there? _____

2. How many pairs of thoracic nerves are there? _____

3. How many pairs of lumbar nerves are there? _____

4. How many pairs of sacral nerves are there? _____

Identification: Figure 5.21 is a diagram of the major parts of the nervous system. Identify the indicated structures by writing the appropriate letter next to the correct term in the space provided.

_____	1. autonomic chain of ganglia	_____	10. peroneal nerve
_____	2. brachial plexus	_____	11. radial nerve
_____	3. brain	_____	12. sacral plexus
_____	4. cervical plexus	_____	13. saphenous nerve
_____	5. femoral nerve	_____	14. sciatic nerve
_____	6. intercostal nerve	_____	15. spinal cord
_____	7. lumbar plexus	_____	16. tibial nerve
_____	8. median nerve	_____	17. ulnar nerve
_____	9. plantar nerve	_____	18. spinal nerve

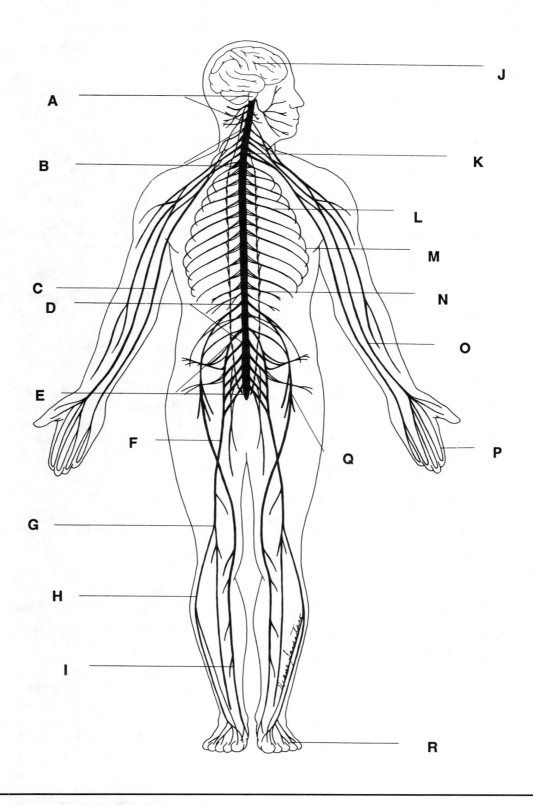

Fig. 5.21   The nervous system.

Key Choices: Choose the key responses that best correspond to the descriptions provided in the following statements. Write the appropriate letter in the space provided.

A. central nervous system   D. autonomic nervous system
B. peripheral nervous system   E. sympathetic nervous system
C. somatic nervous system   F. parasympathetic nervous system

_____ 1. Stimulation causes increased respiration, dilated pupils, increased heart rate, and cardiac output.

_____ 2. Consists of motor nerves, sensory nerves and mixed nerves.

_____ 3. Is completely housed and protected in a bony covering.

_____ 4. General function is to conserve energy.

_____ 5. Is comprised of the sympathetic and parasympathetic nervous system.

_____ 6. Includes the autonomic and somatic nervous system.

_____ 7. Nerve fibers arise from the vagus nerve, the 2nd, 3rd and 4th sacral spinal nerves and the III, VII and IX cranial nerves.

_____ 8. Is composed of cranial nerves, spinal nerves and nerve ganglia.

_____ 9. Is composed of the brain and spinal cord.

_____ 10. Prepares the organism for energy expending, stressful, or emergency situations.

_____ 11. Regulates smooth muscle, the heart, and other involuntary functions.

_____ 12. Interprets incoming information and issues orders.

_____ 13. Carries information to and from all parts of the body.

_____ 14. Carries information to and from the skeletal muscles and skin.

_____ 15. Involves a chain of ganglia located along the spine.

Completion: In the space provided, write the word or words that correctly complete each statement.

1. The simplest form of nervous activity that includes a sensory and motor nerve and few, if any, interneurons is called a _____.

2. The nerve pathway of the simplest form of nervous activity is called a _____.

Identification: Figure 5.22 is a diagram of a simple reflex arc. Identify the indicated structures and write the appropriate letter next to the correct term. Then, draw an arrow to indicate the direction of the nerve impulse.

_____ 1. sensory neuron

_____ 2. dorsal root

_____ 3. motor neuron

_____ 4. intercalated neuron

_____ 5. skin (receptor)

_____ 6. spinal cord

_____ 7. spinal ganglion

_____ 8. ventral root

_____ 9. muscle (effector)

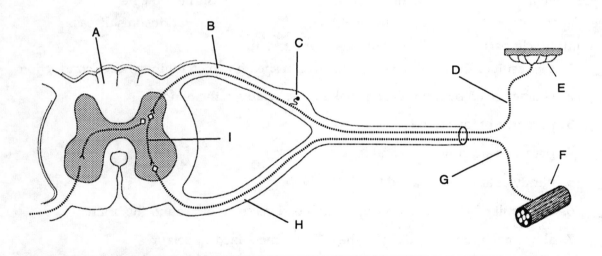

Fig. 5.22   Simple reflex arc.

Completion: In the space provided, write the word or words that correctly complete each statement.

1. Sensory nerves that record conscious sensations such as heat, cold, pain, and pressure are termed _____.

2. Sensory nerves that respond to the unconscious inner sense of position and movement of the body are termed _____.

3. The system of sensory and motor nerve activity that provides information as to the position and rate of movement of different body parts is _____.

4. _____ sense the length and stretch of the muscle as well as how far and fast the muscle is moving.

5. _____ consist of intrafusal muscle fibers, annulo-spiral, and flower-type nerve receptors.

6. _____ are multibranched sensory nerve endings located in tendons in the area where muscle fibers attach to tendon tissue.

7. _____ measure the amount of tension produced in muscle cells that occurs as a result of the muscle stretching and contracting.

Matching: Match the term with the best description. Write the letter of the appropriate term in the space provided.

A. paraplegia   D. quadriplegia   G. hemiplegia

B. epilepsy   E. poliomyelitis   H. Parkinson's disease

C. multiple sclerosis F. cerebrovascular accident

_____ 1. the result of the break down of the myelin sheath, which inhibits nerve conduction

_____ 2. characterized by tremors and shaking, especially in the hands

_____ 3. paralysis of lower body

_____ 4. paralysis affecting arms and legs

_____ 5. paralysis affecting one side of the body

_____ 6. the result of a blood clot or ruptured blood vessel in or around the brain

_____ 7. abnormal electrical activity in the CNS characterized by seizures

_____ 8. a crippling or even deadly disease that affects the motor neurons of the medulla oblongata and spinal cord, resulting in paralysis

Word Review: The student is encouraged to write down the meaning of each of the following words. The list can be used as a study guide for this unit.

afferent nerve	ganglia	parasympathetic nervous system
afferent neuron	golgi tendon organs	peripheral nervous system
arachnoid mater	hemiplegia	pia mater
autonomic nervous system	interneuron	pons
axon	kinesthesia	proprioception
brachial plexus	lumbar plexus	proprioceptors
brain	medulla oblongata	quadriplegia
brain stem	meninges	reflex
central nervous system	midbrain	reflex arc
cerebellum	mixed nerve	sacral plexus
cerebrospinal fluid	motor nerve	sciatic nerve
cerebrovascular accident	motor neuron	sciatica
cerebrum	muscle spindle cells	sensory nerve
cervical plexus	nerve	sensory neuron
cranial nerves	nerve cell	somatic nervous system
dendrite	nerve fibers	spinal cord
dura mater	neuralgia	spinal cord injury
effector	neuritis	stroke
efferent nerve	neuron	sympathetic nervous system
efferent neuron	neurotransmitter	synapse
epilepsy	paraplegia	

System Six: The Endocrine System

Completion: In the space provided, write the word or words that correctly complete each statement.

1. Glands that have tubes or ducts that carry their secretions to a particular part of the body are

   _____ or _____.

2. Glands that depend on the blood and lymph to carry their secretions to various affected tissues are _____ glands.

3. The chemical substances manufactured by the endocrine glands are known as

   _____.

Identification: Figure 5.23 is a diagram of the endocrine glands of the body. In the space provided, write the names of the numbered hormone-producing organ. Also name the hormone-producing organs described in numbers 11,12, and 13.

A.

1. _____   6. _____

2. _____   7. _____

3. _____   8. _____

4. _____   9. _____

5. _____   10. _____

B.

_____ 11. Numbers 5 and 6 hang from the bottom of this hormone-producing organ.

_____ 12. This is only present in pregnant women.

_____ 13. These are the four small glands attached to the thyroid.

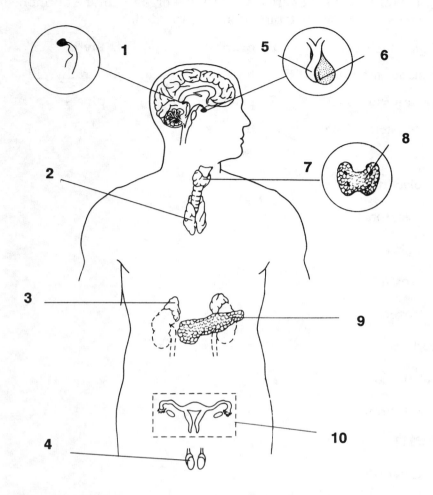

Fig. 5.23   The endocrine system.

Matching: Using the following list of organs, match the organ with the hormone(s) it produces or releases and write the appropriate letter in the space provided.

A. adrenal gland (cortex)   E. ovaries   I. thyroid

B. adrenal gland (medulla)   F. testes   J. parathyroid

C. pituitary (anterior lobe)   G. pancreas   K. pineal

D. pituitary (posterior lobe)   H. thymus

Hormones

_____ 1. prolactin

_____ 2. aldosterone

_____ 3. insulin

_____ 4. thyroxin

_____ 5. estrogen

_____ 6. cortisol

_____ 7. calcitonin

_____ 8. parathormone

_____ 9. ACTH

_____ 10. hydrocortisone

_____ 11. gonadotropic hormones

_____ 12. glucagon

_____ 13. triiodothyronine

_____ 14. oxytocin

_____ 15. progesterone

_____ 16. mineralocorticoids

_____ 17. epinephrine

_____ 18. TSH

_____ 19. testosterone

_____ 20. norepinephrine

_____ 21. growth hormone

_____ 22. corticosteroids

_____ 23. antidiuretic hormone

Matching: Match the term with the best description. Write the letter of the appropriate term next to the best description.

A. adrenocorticotropin   H. insulin
B. aldosterone   I. lactogenic hormone
C. calcitonin   J. luteinizing hormone
D. cortisol   K. oxytocin
E. estrogens   L. parathormone
F. follicle-stimulating hormone   M. progesterone
G. glucagon   N. TSH

_____ 1. antagonistic to insulin, produced by the same gland

_____ 2. promotes the lining of the uterus to thicken in preparation for fertilization

_____ 3. anterior pituitary hormones that regulate the female cycle

_____ 4. stimulates development of secretory parts of mammary glands

_____ 5. directly regulate the menstrual cycle

_____ 6. stimulates thyroid to produce thyroxin

_____ 7. decreases calcium in the blood

_____ 8. increases calcium level in the blood

_____ 9. stimulates mammary glands to secrete milk

_____ 10. helps protect the body during stress; stimulates the adrenal cortex

_____ 11. necessary for glucose to be taken up by cells

Identification: The following list of conditions are usually the result of hyper- or hypoactivity of an endrocine gland's production of a particular hormone. In the first column indicate whether the condition is due to hyper or hypo activity. In the second column write the name of the involved hormone.

_____ _____ 1. giantism

_____ _____ 2. Addison's disease

_____ _____ 3. Graves disease

_____ _____ 4. masculinization; abnormal hairiness

_____ _____ 5. tetany

_____ _____ 6. slow heart rate, sluggish physical and mental activity

_____ _____ 7. spontaneous abortion

_____ _____ 8. acromegaly in an adult

_____ _____ 9. decalcification of bones making them brittle and prone to fracture

_____ _____ 10. high blood glucose; glucose in the urine

_____ _____ 11. Cushing's syndrome

_____ _____ 12. dwarfed stature and mental retardation (cretinism)

_____ _____ 13. failure of the reproductive organs to mature

Word Review: The student is encouraged to write down the meaning of each of the following words. The list can be used as a study guide for this unit.

adrenal glands	goiter	oxytocin
adrenocorticotropic hormone (ACTH)	gonadotropic hormones	pancreas
aldosterone	gonads	parathormone
antidiuretic hormone (ADH)	growth hormone	parathyroid glands
calcitonin	hormones	pituitary gland
cortisol	hyperactive	prolactin
diabetes mellitus	hypoactive	target organs
ducts	hypothalamus	testes
endocrine glands	insulin	testosterone
epinephrine	islets of Langerhans	tetany
estrogen	master gland	thyroid gland
exocrine glands	mineralocorticoids	thyroid stimulating hormone (TSH)
glucagon	norepinephrine	thyroxin
glucocorticoids	ovaries	triiodothyronine

System Seven: The Respiratory System

Identification: Identify the indicated structures in Figure 5.24. Write the correct letters next to the appropriate names in the space provided.

_____ 1. bronchial tree	_____ 6. lungs
_____ 2. roof of mouth	_____ 7. nasal passage
_____ 3. lower jawbone	_____ 8. oral cavity
_____ 4. epiglottis	_____ 9. tongue
_____ 5. larynx	_____ 10. trachea

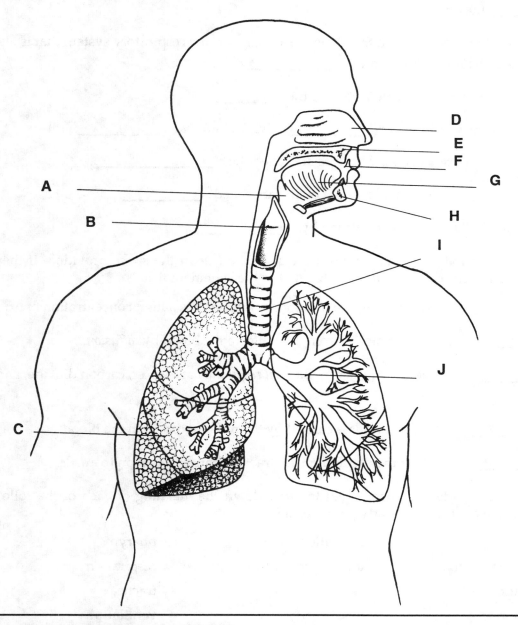

Fig. 5.24   Respiratory organs and structures.

Completion: In the space provided, write the word or words that correctly complete each statement.

1. The exchange of oxygen and carbon dioxide that takes place in the body is called _____.

2. The exchange between the external environment and the blood that takes place in the lungs is termed _____.

3. The gaseous exchange between the blood and the cells of the body is termed _____.

4. The oxidation that occurs within the cell is termed _____.

5. Air enters the nasal cavity through the _____.

6. The function of the mucosa of the nasal cavity is to _____, _____ and _____ the air.

7. The passage way common to the digestive system and the respiratory system that is also referred to as the throat is called the _____.

8. The air passes through the voice box or the _____.

9. In the chest the wind pipe or _____ divides into two _____.

10. The entire multibranched air passages are called the _____.

11. The air passages terminate in clusters of air sacs called _____.

12. The act of ventilation is accomplished by _____.

True or False: If the following statements are true, write *true* in the space provided. If they are false, replace the italicized word with one that makes the statement true.

_____ 1. The blood in the pulmonary arteries has a high concentration of *oxygen*.

_____ 2. Oxygen moves from the lungs to the blood by *diffusion*.

_____ 3. The by-products of *internal respiration* are water, carbon dioxide, and energy.

_____ 4. *Carbon dioxide* is carried by the red blood cells in the blood.

_____ 5. When the diaphragm contracts, it causes a person to *exhale*.

Word Review: The student is encouraged to write down the meaning of each of the following words. The list can be used as a study guide for this unit.

alveoli	inhalation	pharynx
cellular respiration	internal respiration	respiration
diaphragm	larynx	trachea
exhalation	nasal cavity	ventilation
external respiration	oxidation	

System Eight: The Digestive System

Completion: In the space provided, write the word or words that correctly complete each statement.

1. The process of converting food into substances capable of nourishing cells is _____.

2. The process in which the digested nutrients are transferred from the intestines to the blood or lymph vessels to be transported to the cells is _____.

3. The muscular tube that goes from the lips to the anus is the _____ or the _____.

4. Organs that aid digestion but are located outside the digestive tract are known as _____ digestive organs.

5. The physical activity of digestion that takes place in the mouth is _____.

6. The chemical digestive activity that takes place in the mouth is from secretions by the _____.

7. The physical or mechanical activity in the alimentary canal is from the action of the _____.

Identification: Identify the indicated structures in Figure 5.25. Write the correct names next to the appropriate numbers in the space provided.

1. _____   7. _____
2. _____   8. _____
3. _____   9. _____
4. _____   10. _____
5. _____   11. _____
6. _____   12. _____

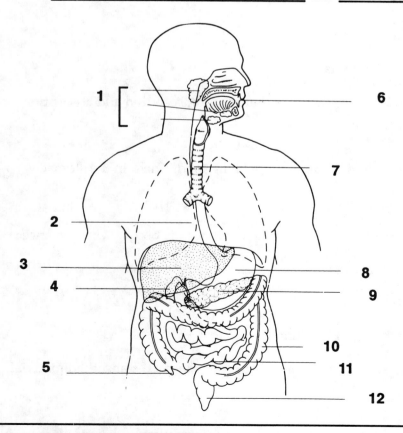

Fig. 5.25   The digestive system.

Matching: Match the term with the best description. Write the letter of the appropriate term in the space provided.

A. bolus	G. ileocecal valve	M. pyloric valve
B. cardiac sphincter	H. ileum	N. rectum
C. cecum	I. lacteals	O. saliva
D. chyme	J. mucosa	P. serous layer
E. colon	K. oral cavity	Q. submucosa
F. duodenum	L. peristalsis	R. villa

_____ 1. beginning of the large intestine

_____ 2. contains enzymes that begin to break down carbohydrates

_____ 3. a mixture of digestive juices, mucous, and food material

_____ 4. a soft food ball that is swallowed

_____ 5. prevents movement from the large intestine to the small intestine

_____ 6. outer covering of the tube that is continuous with the peritoneum lining the abdominal cavity

_____ 7. rhythmic, wavelike, muscular motion

_____ 8. opening at the top of the stomach

_____ 9. temporary storage of solid waste

_____ 10. opening at the end of the stomach

_____ 11. a membrane made up of epithelial cells that carry on secretion and absorption

_____ 12. where food is masticated

_____ 13. plays an important role in determining how long food is held in the stomach

_____ 14. first section of small intestine

_____ 15. stores, forms, and excretes waste products; regulates the body's water balance

_____ 16. fingerlike projections that increase surface area of small intestines

_____ 17. organ that receives bile and pancreatic juices

_____ 18. lymph capillaries in the small intestine

_____ 19. serves to nourish the surrounding tissues and carry away the absorbed material

_____ 20. last section of small intestine

_____ 21. organ responsible for water absorption and feces formation

Word Review: The student is encouraged to write down the meaning of each of the following words. The list can be used as a study guide for this unit.

absorption	descending colon	pancreatic fluid
accessory digestive organs	digestion	peristalsis
alimentary canal	duodenum	pyloric sphincter
anal canal	feces	rectum
ascending colon	hydrochloric acid	saliva
bile	ileum	salivary glands
bolus	ileocecal valve	sigmoid colon
cardiac sphincter	intestinal digestive juices	small intestine
cecum	jejunum	transverse colon
chyme	lacteals	villi
colon	oral cavity	
common bile duct	pancreatic duct	

System Nine: The Excretory System

Matching: Match the term with the best description. Write the letter or letters of the appropriate excretory organ next to the term describing what that organ eliminates.

A. kidneys   C. liver   E. skin

B. large intestine   D. lungs

_____ 1. urine

_____ 2. food wastes

_____ 3. expiration

_____ 4. bile

_____ 5. uric acid

_____ 6. feces

_____ 7. urea

_____ 8. heat

_____ 9. CO_2

_____ 10. perspiration

_____ 11. water

Completion: In the space provided, write the word or words that correctly complete each statement.

1. The functional unit of the kidney is the _____.

2. The tubes that carry urine from the kidneys to the bladder are called _____.

3. A hormone produced in the kidneys that acts to regulate blood pressure is _____.

True or False: If the following statements are true, write *true* in the space provided. If they are false, replace the italicized word with one that makes the statement true.

_____ 1. The kidneys normally filter forty to fifty *gallons* of blood plasma a day.

_____ 2. When a person urinates, *voluntary* muscles in the walls of the bladder contract forcing the urine out of the body.

Identification: Identify the indicated structures in Figure 5.26. Write the correct names next to the appropriate numbers in the space provided.

1. _____   6. _____

2. _____   7. _____

3. _____   8. _____

4. _____   9. _____

5. _____   10. _____

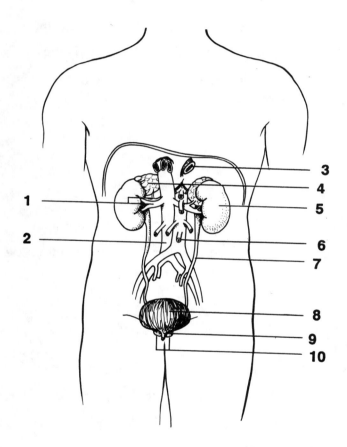

Fig. 5.26   The urinary system.

Word Review: The student is encouraged to write down the meaning of each of the following words. The list can be used as a study guide for this unit.

bile	metabolic wastes	ureters
bladder	nephron	urethra
excretion	renin	urinary system

System Ten: The Human Reproductive System

Completion: In the space provided, write the word or words that correctly complete each statement.

1. One-celled organisms that do not need a partner to reproduce do so by nonsexual means called _____ reproduction.

2. The term used to describe a reproductive cell that can unite with another reproductive cell to form the cell that develops into a new individual is called a _____.

3. In males, the reproductive cells are called _____.

4. In females, the reproductive cells are called _____.

5. The cell formed by the union of the male and female reproductive cells is called a _____.

6. The gland in the female that produces the reproductive cell is the _____.

7. The gland in the male that produces the reproductive cell is the _____.

Short Answer: Number the following terms from 1 to 5 in the order that sperm would travel from the time it is produced until it leaves the body.

_____ vas deferens

_____ urethra

_____ epididymis

_____ seminiferous tubules

_____ ejaculatory ducts

Matching: Match the term with the best description. Write the letter of the appropriate term next to the best description.

A. Cowper's glands   E. testes
B. epididymis   F. urethra
C. prostate gland   G. vas deferens
D. seminal vesicles

_____ 1. conveys both urine and sperm out of the body

_____ 2. two convoluted, glandular tubes located on each side of the prostate gland

_____ 3. stores the sperm until it becomes fully mature

_____ 4. forms the male hormone testosterone

_____ 5. mucus producing glands that serve to lubricate the urethra

_____ 6. contains specialized cells that produce the spermatozoa

_____ 7. surrounds the first part of the urethra

_____ 8. two pea-sized glands located beneath the prostate gland

_____ 9. secrets an alkaline fluid that neutralizes the acidic vaginal secretions

_____ 10. secretions contain simple sugars, mucus, prostaglandin

_____ 11. two small, egg-shaped glands made up of minute convoluted tubules

_____ 12. sperm collects here until it is expelled from the body

_____ 13. located in the scrotum; receives sperm from the testes

Identification: Identify the indicated structures in Figure 5.27. Write the correct letter next to the appropriate name in the space provided.

_____ 1. bulbourethral gland

_____ 2. ejaculation duct

_____ 3. epididymis

_____ 4. erectile tissue

_____ 5. glans penis

_____ 6. prepuce

_____ 7. prostate gland

_____ 8. scrotum

_____ 9. seminal vesicle

_____ 10. seminiferous tubules

_____ 11. testis

_____ 12. urinary bladder

_____ 13. vas deferens

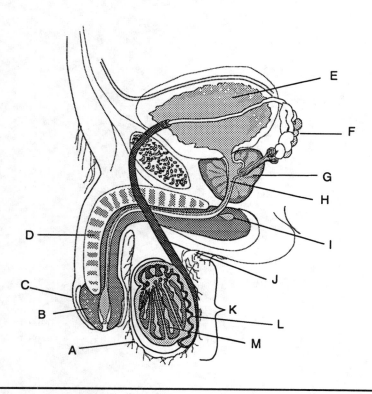

Fig. 5.27   The male reproductive system.

Completion: In the space provided, write the word or words that correctly complete each statement.

1. The external part of the female reproductive system that includes the labia majora and the labia minora is termed the _____.

2. The muscular tube or canal that is the lower part of the birth canal is called the _____.

3. The chamber that houses the developing fetus is the _____.

4. The egg-carrying tubes of the female reproductive system are the _____.

5. The glands that produce estrogen and progesterone are the _____.

6. The egg cell capable of being fertilized by a spermatozoon is the _____.

Identification: Identify the indicated structures in Figure 5.28. Write the correct letter next to the appropriate terms in the space provided.

_____ 1. anal opening

_____ 2. cervix

_____ 3. fimbrae

_____ 4. fallopian tube

_____ 5. labium minora

_____ 6. labium majora

_____ 7. ovary

_____ 8. spine

_____ 9. rectum

_____ 10. symphysis pubis

_____ 11. urethra

_____ 12. urinary bladder

_____ 13. uterus

_____ 14. vagina

_____ 15. urinary opening

_____ 16. fundus of uterus

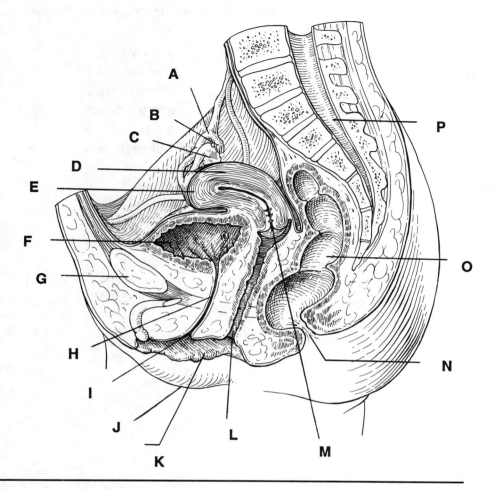

Fig. 5.28   The female reproductive system.

Matching: Match the term with the best description. Write the letter of the appropriate term in the space provided.

A. corpus luteum   C. gestation   E. menstruation

B. estrogen   D. menopause   F. ovulation

_____ 1. controls the development of secondary female sexual characteristics

_____ 2. the release of the egg cell from the ovary

_____ 3. ovarian site of estrogen and progesterone production

_____ 4. occurs from the time an ovum is fertilized until childbirth

_____ 5. the cyclic uterine bleeding that normally occurs at about four week intervals

_____ 6. follicle transformed by luteinizing hormone

_____ 7. the physiological cessation of the menstrual cycle

Word Review: The student is encouraged to write down the meaning of each of the following words. The list can be used as a study guide for this unit.

asexual reproduction	labia minora	semen
bulbourethral glands	luteinizing hormone	seminal fluid
cervix	menopause	seminal vesicles
corpus luteum	menstrual cycle	spermatozoa
ejaculatory ducts	menstruation	testes
epididymis	penis	testosterone
estrogen	pregnancy	urethra
fallopian tubes	ovary	uterus
fertilization	oviducts	vagina
fetus	ovulation	vas deferens
gamete	ovum	vulva
gestation	progesterone	zygote
gonad	prostate gland	
labia majora	scrotum	

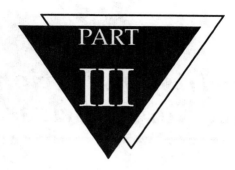

Massage Practice

Effects, Benefits, Indications, and Contraindications of Massage

Completion: In the space provided, write the word or words that correctly complete each statement.

1. A massage should not be given when _____ are present.

2. Direct physical effects of the massage techniques on the tissues are considered to be _____ effects.

3. Indirect responses to touch that affect body functions and tissues through the nervous or energy systems are termed _____ effects.

4. Effects of massage on the structures of the body are considered _____ effects.

5. Mental and emotional effects of massage are _____ effects.

6. An existing condition that renders a massage or treatment to all or part of the body inadvisable is a _____.

True or False: If the following statements are true, write *true* in the space provided. If they are false, replace the italicized word with one that makes the statement true.

_____ 1. Kneading and compression help to increase *strength* in muscles.

_____ 2. *Active joint movements* increase strength, flexibility, and circulation.

Matching: Select the massage technique that is best described by the phrase. Place the letter(s) next to the appropriate description in the space provided.

A. active joint movements   D. friction   G. passive joint movement

B. compression   E. kneading   H. percussion

C. deep stroking   F. light stroking   I. vibration

_____ 1. prevents and reduces excessive scarring following trauma

_____ 2. rotation of joints through their range of motion with no resistance or assistance by muscular activity on the part of the client

_____ 3. relaxes and lengthens the muscles

_____ 4. prevents and reduces the development of adhesions

_____ 5. contraction of voluntary muscles are by the client, either resisted or assisted by the therapist

_____ 6. helps to firm and strengthen muscles

_____ 7. produces calming sedative effects

_____ 8. directed toward the heart in the direction of venous blood flow

_____ 9. increases the permeability of the capillary beds and produces an increased flow of interstitial fluid

_____ 10. produces a hyperemia in the muscle tissue

Matching: Select the most appropriate answer(s) from the choices given. Write the letter(s) of the choice next to the appropriate description in the space provided.

    A. Avoid the affected area.

    B. Consult with the client's physician before proceeding.

    C. Do not perform the massage at this time.

    D. Massage specifically on the affected area.

    E. Proceed with a light noninvasive, soothing massage.

    F. Proceed with the massage as usual.

    G. Refer the client to a doctor.

_____ 1. Miss Harris is twenty-six years old and has been in to see you on a monthly basis. When she comes in for her regular appointment, she complains of a general achiness, is slightly flushed, and has a temperature of 101.5 degrees.

_____ 2. Mrs. Clements asks for you to come to her home to give her a massage. She says she would come to your office except that she has the flu.

_____ 3. Mr. James's wrist is red, swollen, and warm to the touch. He has come in for a general massage and asks you to pay particular attention to his wrist.

_____ 4. Mrs. Annest has come in for a massage. As she is getting on the table, you notice a red, flaky area on the inside of her elbow and another one on the back of her shoulder. When you ask, she says that they are "just some itchy patches she has had for a couple of weeks."

_____ 5. When Mr. Inkles lies face down on the table, you notice a number inflamed bumps and pimples between his shoulder blades and on his shoulders.

_____ 6. Mr. Johnson, a forty-year-old, indicates that he is under a doctor's care for a condition that has caused a severe decalcification of the bones.

_____ 7. An eighty-three-year-old woman with noticeably stoop shoulders, and somewhat deformed hands wants to start getting massages to help recover from a fractured hip she suffered three months ago.

_____ 8. A thirty-five-year-old mother of three comes in for relief of sore feet and an achy lower back. When giving her a massage, you notice several bulging bluish masses on her legs.

_____ 9. A twenty-eight-year-old man comes into the clinic for a massage. He says that he was thrown from a horse two days before and has a lot of discomfort in his hip and thigh. When he gets on the table, you note a large black and blue area around his hip. He says he has gone to the doctor and x-rays determined there were no broken bones.

_____ 10. A thirty-five-year-old woman comes in for a massage. One week earlier she was in a car accident. No bones were broken, but she was shaken up pretty badly. She has large bruises on her upper arm and thigh that are still somewhat discolored.

_____ 11. A woman who is seven months pregnant comes in and wants a massage because she is "stressed out." You notice that her hands and feet are somewhat swollen. When you press a finger into her ankle, it leaves a slight impression.

_____ 12. Mr. Hill is fifty-four years old and is under a physician's care for high blood pressure. His physician has recommended massage as part of his treatment. You take his blood pressure when he comes for his massage and it is 170 over 130.

_____ 13. Mrs. Baird is forty-four years old and is in the middle of a series of chemotherapy treatments after having a malignant growth removed from her colon. She is seeking massage for relief from stress and "to be good to herself."

_____ 14. A forty-eight-year-old female executive is under a doctor's care for chronic fatigue and mental exhaustion. The doctor has recommended massage as part of her treatment.

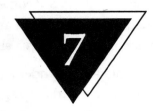

Equipment and Products

Completion: In the space provided, write the word or words that correctly complete each statement.

1. Professionalism is an _____.

2. As a massage practitioner, list at least four ways to project a professional image.

   a. _____   c. _____

   b. _____   d. _____

3. When operating a massage facility, two standards that must be maintained are _____ and _____.

4. The optimum temperature for a massage room is _____.

5. To assure an abundant supply of fresh air, a massage room should have good
   _____.

6. The lighting in a massage room should be _____.

7. A massage practitioner's most important piece of equipment is the _____.

8. Three attributes of a good massage table are that it is _____ and
   _____.

9. In order to give the practitioner leverage and to prevent fatigue, the massage table must be
   _____.

10. A good width for a massage table is _____.

11. A good length for a massage table is _____.

12. One of a massage practitioner's most important supplies is the _____ they use on their clients.

13. If there is reason to believe the client is sensitive or allergic to a product or oil, the practitioner can perform a _____.

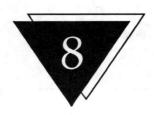

Sanitary and Safety Practices

Completion: In the space provided, write the word or words that correctly complete each statement.

1. In personal care services, public health is protected by _____ and _____.

2. The removal of microorganisms is _____.

3. Any item that comes in contact with the client must be clean and _____.

4. A massage practitioner's hands can be sanitized by _____.

5. Minute, unicellular microorganisms exhibiting both plant and animal characteristics are called _____.

6. Beneficial and harmless bacteria that perform useful functions are termed _____.

7. Bacteria that cause or produce disease are termed _____.

8. Three general forms of pathogenic bacteria are _____, _____ and _____.

9. The body's natural ability to resist infection is _____.

10. The body's most important defense against invasion of harmful bacteria is the _____.

11. A class of proteins produced in the body in response to contact with an invading bacteria is an _____.

12. Microscopic pathogenic agents that invade living cells and are capable of transmitting disease are called _____.

13. The primary precaution in infection control is thorough _____.

14. An acceptable way to sanitize linens is to wash them in _____ water and add one-fourth to one-half cup of _____.

15. Floors, sinks, and restrooms can be cleaned and sanitized with a solution of _____.

16. The practitioner's hands can be sanitized by _____.

17. If there is suspicion of bacterial contamination, the hands can be rinsed with _____.

Short Answer: In the space provided, write a short answer to the following questions.

1. If a client has an infection or contagious disease, what are two things the massage practitioner should do?

   a. _____

   b. _____

2. When should the massage practitioner wash their hands?

   _____

3. List three acceptable means of sanitizing implements.

   a. _____

   b. _____

   c. _____

4. List three agents that can be used to disinfect implements.

   a. _____

   b. _____

   c. _____

Matching: Match the methods of disinfecting or sterilization with the given situation. Write the letter or letters of the appropriate procedure in the space provided.

A. boiling in water   F. rinsing with formalin solution

B. chlorine bleach   G. rinsing with alcohol solution

C. creosol or Lysol   H. soap and hot water

D. immersing in quats   I. wiping with alcohol

E. immersing in formalin

_____ 1. massage table surface with normal use

_____ 2. massage table face cradle

_____ 3. practitioner's hands before a massage

_____ 4. practitioner's hands after a massage

_____ 5. practitioner's hands after working on client with possible contagious skin condition

_____ 6. bathroom sink

_____ 7. bathroom floor

_____ 8. shower stall

_____ 9. linens after normal use

_____ 10. linens after use on client with possible contagious condition

_____ 11. brushes and combs kept for client use

_____ 12. towels used for wraps and hydrotherapy

_____ 13. fever thermometer before use

_____ 14. fever thermometer after use

The Consultation

Completion: In the space provided, write the word or words that correctly complete each statement.

1. A meeting between the prospective client and the practitioner where views are discussed and valuable information is exchanged is called a _____.

2. In order for a consultation to be effective, there must be clear _____ between the client and the practitioner.

3. The two most effective ways for the practitioner to ask questions of the client are _____ and _____.

Short Answer: In the space provided, write a short answer to the following questions.

1. List six things the therapist can accomplish during the consultation.

    a. _____

    b. _____

    c. _____

    d. _____

    e. _____

    f. _____

2. When making a first appointment with a prospective client, what are three questions that can be asked in order to screen them?

    a. _____

    b. _____

    c. _____

3. List four areas that a practitioner may include in a policy statement.

    a. _____

    b. _____

    c. _____

    d. _____

4. Three reasons to perform a preliminary assessment are to:

    a. _____

    b. _____

    c. _____

Completion: In the space provided, write the word or words that correctly complete each statement.

1. To help disclose problems and the physiological basis for the client's complaints, an assessment includes _____, _____ and _____.

2. Information gained from intake and medical forms, answers to questions, and descriptions the client offers are the basis for the _____.

3. Noticing how clients hold their bodies, how they move, and how they react to questions or manipulative tests is part of _____.

4. Various manipulative and verbal tests that help determine more precisely the tissues or conditions involved are part of the _____.

5. The outline a practitioner develops and follows when giving massage treatments is termed a _____.

Short Answer: In the space provided, write a short answer to the following questions.

1. List four sources of information used when formulating a treatment plan.

    a. _____

    b. _____

    c. _____

    d. _____

2. List the kind of information that is kept in the client files.

    a. _____

    b. _____

    c. _____

    d. _____

3. What information does a practitioner record in a treatment record?

    a. _____

    b. _____

    c. _____

    d. _____

    e. _____

    f. _____

Completion: In the space provided, write the word or words that correctly complete each statement.

1. During a consultation, if the client appears flushed, unusually warm, and does not feel well, then it is best to take his or her _____ and _____.

2. A marked elevation in body temperature tends to increase the _____.

3. The average resting pulse rate of an adult is between _____ beats per minute.

4. The pulse rate is the number of beats counted in _____ seconds and multiplied by 4 (or 60 seconds).

5. The most common area to palpate for the pulse is the _____.

6. Normal temperature is about _____.

7. An abnormally high pulse or body temperature is a _____ for massage.

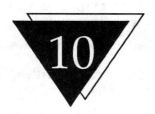

Classification of Massage Movements

Completion: In the space provided, write the word or words that correctly complete each statement.

1. Three physical factors that control the results of a manipulation are the _____, _____ and _____ of the movement.

2. Another important factor that affects the outcome of a technique or massage is the _____ with which it is given.

3. In Swedish massage most movements are directed _____ the heart.

4. Massage strokes are directed toward the heart in order to affect the flow of _____ and _____.

5. The six major categories of massage movements are _____, _____, _____, _____, _____ and _____.

Identification: Name the classification of massage manipulation described in each statement. Write the correct classification next to the appropriate description in the space provided.

_____ 1. applied in the direction of the venous and lymphatic flow

_____ 2. lifts, squeezes, and presses the tissues

_____ 3. used to distribute any lubricant and to prepare the area for other techniques

_____ 4. manipulation of the articulations of the client

_____ 5. generally the first and last contact the practitioner has with the client

_____ 6. placing of the practitioner's hand or fingers on the client without movement in any direction

_____ 7. rapid striking motion against the surface of the client's body

_____ 8. moving more superficial layers of flesh against the deeper tissues

_____ 9. moving a body part through a range of motion

_____ 10. the stationary contact of the practitioner's hand and the client's body

_____ 11. moving the hand over some portion of the client's body with varying amounts of pressure

_____ 12. used to assist a client to restore mobility or increase flexibility in a joint

105

_____ 13. raising tissues from their ordinary position and then squeezing, rolling, or pinching with firm pressure

_____ 14. manipulating one layer of tissue over or against another

Matching: Touch and gliding techniques can be further classified as superficial or deep. In the space provided write the letter or letters of the most appropriate technique next to the description.

    A. superficial touch   C. superficial gliding

    B. deep touch   D. deep gliding

_____ 1. Client has moderately high blood pressure.

_____ 2. Client is nervous and irritated.

_____ 3. Client is in pain from severe arthritis.

_____ 4. Client is healthy with thick, heavy musculature.

_____ 5. Client has trigger points in the neck and shoulders.

_____ 6. Client is critically ill with lymphoma.

_____ 7. Client has stress points in the tendons around the elbow and knee.

_____ 8. Client complains of insomnia.

_____ 9. This is the main technique used in foot reflexology.

_____ 10. This technique is used when applying oil to the body.

_____ 11. Client requests a deep relaxing massage.

_____ 12. This is the main technique used in shiatzu.

_____ 13. Client is generally tired and mildly fatigued.

_____ 14. Client is visibly nervous and tense.

Matching: Match the terms with the best description. Write the letter of the best description in the space provided.

_____ 1. hacking

_____ 2. skin rolling

_____ 3. aura stroking

_____ 4. active, assistive joint movements

_____ 5. superficial gliding

_____ 6. cross fiber friction

_____ 7. kneading

_____ 8. friction

_____ 9. superficial touch

_____ 10. circular friction

_____ 11. tapping

_____ 12. active, resistive joint movements

_____ 13. feather stroking

A. rhythmic pumping action directed into the muscle perpendicular to the body part

B. a stroke with enough pressure to have a mechanical effect

C. applied in a transverse direction across the muscle, tendon, or ligament fibers

D. the natural weight of the practitioner's finger, fingers, or hand held on a given area of the client's body.

E. quick, striking manipulations with ulnar border of the hand

F. help from the practitioner as the client moves a limb

G. moving the skin in a circular pattern over the deeper tissues

_____ 14. compression

_____ 15. deep touch

_____ 16. passive joint
movements

_____ 17. deep gliding

_____ 18. vibration

H. a continuous shaking or trembling movement transmitted from the practitioner's hand or an electrical appliance

I. very light fingertip pressure with long, flowing strokes

J. moving more superficial layers of flesh against deeper tissues

K. applying pressure with no other movement

L. picking the skin and subcutaneous tissue up between the thumbs and fingers and rolling

M. moving a flexible, firm hand lightly over extended area of the body.

N. raising the skin and muscular tissues from their ordinary position and squeezing with a firm pressure, usually in a circular direction

O. quick, striking manipulations with tips of the fingers

P. moving a client's joint while their muscles are relaxed

Q. the practitioner's resistance of a client's movement

R. hands gliding over a body part without touching

True or False: If the following statements are true, write _true_ in the space provided. If they are false, replace the italicized word with one that makes the statement true.

_____ 1. Massage strokes directed away from the heart are termed _centripetal_.

_____ 2. In order to have a _sedating_ effect, the rhythm of the massage must be steady and slightly faster than the client's natural rhythm.

_____ 3. A primary indication of tension and dysfunction in soft tissue is _numbness_.

_____ 4. The pressure used with a massage technique should start out light, then increase and end _light_.

_____ 5. Deep massage techniques that cause a client to react in pain must be _avoided_.

Application of Massage Technique

Completion: In the space provided, write the word or words that correctly complete each statement.

1. The primary tools the practitioner uses when giving a massage are the _____.

2. The practitioner conserves energy and increases power in massage movements by using his or her _____.

3. The observation of body postures in relation to safe and efficient body movement is called _____.

4. To increase strength and power and at the same time reduce the chance of fatigue and injury, the practitioner must use _____.

5. The risk of injury to the body is directly proportionate to the amount of stress and the amount of _____.

6. The Chinese term for the body's geographical center is the _____.

7. The state of self assurance, balance, and emotional stability is often referred to as being _____.

8. The concept that the practitioner functions as a conduit or conductor allowing negative energies to pass out of the client and positive energies to flow in is known as _____.

9. The most common stances for the practitioner while performing a massage are called _____.

10. The stance in which both feet are placed in line with the edge of the table is called the _____.

11. The most commonly used stance is _____.

12. An exercise that helps the practitioner reach the full length of a client's body part while shifting weight on the feet and maintaining good posture and balance is called _____.

13. An exercise in which one imagines turning a large wheel is called _____.

14. An exercise that involves a powerful forward movement followed by a controlled withdrawal is called _____.

15. The exercise that emphasizes the importance of posture, concentration, centering, grounding, and correct breathing is called _____.

Short Answer: Write short answers to the following questions or statements in the spaces provided.

1. When practicing most massage techniques, where should the practitioner's hands be?

    _____

2. In what way does the practitioner apply deeper pressure or more force to a movement?

    _____

3. Why is it important to the practitioner not to raise and tighten the shoulders when giving a massage?

    _____

4. List seven advantages of using good body mechanics and proper stances when giving massages.

    a. _____

    _____

    b. _____

    c. _____

    _____

    d. _____

    e. _____

    _____

    f. _____

    _____

    g. _____

Short Answer: Provide short answers to the following questions. Write your answers in the space provided.

1. What are two important objectives of a good massage sequence?

    a. _____

    b. _____

2. When considering a sequence for a full body massage, what are two primary considerations?

    a. _____

    b. _____

3. Arrange the following body parts into a sequence for a massage. Begin with the right hand and successively number the body parts in the order they would be massaged.

_____ back   _____ neck (face up)

_____ face   _____ right arm

_____ left arm   _____ right foot

_____ left foot   _____ right hand

_____ left hand   _____ right leg (back)

_____ left leg (back)   _____ right leg (front)

_____ left leg (front)   _____ torso

4. Arrange the following body parts into a sequence for a massage. Begin with the left foot and successively number the body parts in the order they would be massaged.

_____ back   _____ right hand

_____ left arm   _____ right arm

_____ left foot   _____ right foot

_____ left hand   _____ right leg (back)

_____ left leg (back)   _____ right leg (front)

_____ left leg (front)   _____ torso

_____ neck (face up)

5. **A.** Arrange the following body parts into a sequence for a massage of the front of the body. Begin with the face and finish the front of the body by massaging the torso. Successively number the body parts in the order they would be massaged.

_____ face   _____ right arm

_____ left arm   _____ right foot

_____ left foot   _____ right hand

_____ left hand   _____ right leg

_____ left leg   _____ torso

_____ neck

B. Alternate the sequence if the right arm is done first.

_____ face	_____ right arm
_____ left arm	_____ right foot
_____ left foot	_____ right hand
_____ left hand	_____ right leg
_____ left leg	_____ torso
_____ neck	

Key Choices: In the following sequence of movements for a body part, fill in the spaces with the most appropriate choices from the following list of movements.

effleurage	friction movements	petrissage
feather strokes	joint movements	

1. applying the oil

2. _____

3. _____

4. effleurage

5. _____

6. effleurage

7. _____

8. effleurage

9. _____

10. redraping

Short Answer: Provide short answers to the following questions. Write your answers in the space provided.

1. When should the practitioner wash their hands?

    _____

2. List four ways to avoid chilling the client.

    a. _____

    b. _____

    c. _____

    d. _____

3. In what direction should gliding movements be given?

    _____

4. Why should extremely heavy or jarring movements be avoided?

    _____

Procedures for Complete Body Massages

Short Answer: Provide short answers to the following questions. Write your answers in the space provided.

1. What is the purpose of explaining your general procedures to clients on their first visit?

   a. _____

   b. _____

2. Ideally, what clothing should a client wear when getting a massage?

   _____

3. How can the practitioner dispel anxiety the client may have about nudity?

   _____

   _____

4. Why should the practitioner assist the client on and off of the table?

   _____

5. How can the practitioner assure that the client assumes the correct position on the table?

   _____

6. What can be done if a client cannot lie down for a massage?

   _____

Completion: In the space provided, write the word or words that correctly complete each statement.

1. The procedure used to assure a client's warmth and sense of modesty is called _____.

2. The implement used to support a client who cannot comfortably lie flat on the table is a _____.

3. The process of using linens to keep a client covered while performing a massage is called _____.

Short Answer: Provide short answers to the following questions. Write your answers in the space provided.

1. What are three advantages of draping to clients?

    a. _____

    b. _____

    c. _____

2. What advantage does draping offer the practitioner?

    _____

    _____

3. What is a good temperature for a massage room?

    _____

4. For those times when the massage room is slightly cool, name two things the practitioner can use to assure the client's warmth.

    a. _____

    b. _____

5. When using proper draping procedures, what part of the client's body is uncovered?

    _____

6. List three types of draping and the linens required for each.

    a. _____

    b. _____

    c. _____

Short Answer: Provide short answers to the following questions. Write your answers in the space provided.

1. In order to get from the dressing area or hydrotherapy area to the massage table, what covering does the client use to maintain modesty:

    a. when using the diaper draping method?

    _____

    b. when using top sheet draping?

    _____

    c. when using single sheet draping?

    _____

Short Answer: Provide short answers to the following questions. Write your answers in the space provided.

1. The client uses a wrap or towel to get from the dressing area to the massage table. What size should it be?

   _____

   _____

2. Where should the opening on the wrap be located?

   _____

3. List three reasons it is important to maintain contact with the client once it is established.

   a. _____

   _____

   b. _____

   _____

   c. _____

   _____

Short Answer: Provide short answers to the following questions. Write your answers in the space provided.

1. In Swedish style massage an oil or lubricant is used. Describe the three-step procedure for applying the lubricant from its container to the client's body?

   a. _____

   b. _____

   _____

   c. _____

   _____

2. How is contact with the client maintained when preparing to apply a lubricant?

   _____

   _____

3. What massage strokes are directed toward the heart?

   _____

4. What strokes can be directed away from the heart?

   _____

5. Why are strokes directed toward the heart?

_____

6. What part of the hand is used to apply gliding strokes to larger areas of the body?

_____

7. Why follow deep friction movements with gliding strokes?

_____

8. What is the first massage technique used after the oil is applied to a body part?

_____

9. What preliminary steps should be taken before a client arrives for a massage?

_____

_____

10. How should the client be greeted?

_____

11. When should an information form be filled out?

_____

Short Answer: Provide short answers to the following questions. Write your answers in the space provided.

1. Name three areas of the body where lubricant is usually not needed?

_____

2. Why are gliding strokes repeated between other massage strokes?

_____

3. How many gliding strokes are usually applied between other strokes in a general massage?

_____

4. When applying gliding strokes to the arm, in which direction is pressure applied?

_____

5. When applying long gliding strokes to the leg with both hands, which hand leads?

_____

6. What does the acronym ASIS stand for?

_____

7. When extending the leg during joint movements, why is it important to keep one hand behind the knee?

_____

8. What is the massage technique most likely to increase muscle length and increase range of motion?

_____

9. What special consideration must be given when massaging a woman's torso?

_____

10. When working on the abdomen, what is the general direction of the massage movements?

_____

11. What is the "caring stroke?"

_____

12. What are the lightest gliding strokes using only the finger tips?

_____

Short Answer: Provide short answers to the following questions. Write your answers in the space provided.

1. Why is a client encouraged to drink plenty of water following massage?

_____

2. How much water is suggested to drink per day?

_____

3. Client's sometimes feel adverse aftereffects following massage. What are four possible adverse aftereffects?

   a. _____

   b. _____

   c. _____

   d. _____

4. What is thought to be the cause of these side effects?

_____

Completion: In the space provided, write the word or words that correctly complete each statement.

1. The four steps of a therapeutic procedure are _____ _____ _____ and _____.

2. Reviewing any information available at the onset of the process takes place during the _____ stage of the therapeutic procedure.

3. Determining strategies and selecting therapeutic techniques to address specific conditions takes place during the _____ stage of the therapeutic procedure.

4. Examining the outcome of the session in regard to the effectiveness of the selected procedure for the condition takes place during the _____ stage of the therapeutic procedure.

5. Recording the client history, examination, and observation takes place during the _____ stage of the therapeutic procedure.

Short Answer: Provide short answers to the following questions. Write your answers in the space provided.

1. What are two methods of obtaining a client history?

_____

2. When does the observation portion of an assessment begin?

_____

3. What are three things a therapist can watch for while observing a client?

a. _____

b. _____

c. _____

4. During the observation phase of an assessment, what does bilateral symmetry refer to?

_____

Completion: In the space provided, write the word or words that correctly complete each statement.

1. Structural deviations, such as a tilted head, rotated hips, or a raised shoulder, are often the result of _____.

2. Posture is best observed when a person is _____ and is best done from _____ sides.

3. The action of a joint through the entire extent of its movement is called _____.

4. Three modes used in assessing the quality of this movement are _____, _____, and _____ movement.

5. The English osteopath who developed a system of testing joints and soft tissue lesions was _____.

6. According to his definition, fibrous tissues that have tensions placed on them during muscular contractions are called _____.

7. Tissues that are not contractile, such as bone, ligament, bursa, blood vessels, nerves, nerve coverings, and cartilage, are _____.

8. The quality of the sensation the therapist feels as they passively move a joint to the full extent of its possible range is termed _____.

9. The results of testing that the therapist is able to see or feel are called _____.

10. The results of tests that the client feels, such as pain or discomfort, and the way the client reacts to the discomfort are considered to be _____ findings.

11. When assessing _____ movement, the client moves through a particular range of motion totally unassisted.

12. It is termed _____ when the practitioner moves the client's joint through full range of motion while the client remains relaxed.

Short Answer: Provide short answers to the following questions. Write your answers in the space provided.

1. When testing range of motion, which side should be tested first?

    _____

2. In what order should the three modes of testing range of motion be performed?

    a. _____

    b. _____

    c. _____

3. What tissues are involved during active movement?

    _____

4. If there is pain during active movement, what are four things the therapist should note?

    a. _____

    b. _____

    c. _____

    d. _____

5. If there is a limitation to the movement during active movement, what are two things the therapist should note?

    a. _____

    b. _____

Completion: In the space provided, write the word or words that correctly complete each statement.

1. There are three types of end feel considered normal. An abrupt, painless limitation to further movement that happens at the normal end of the range of motion, such as knee or elbow extension, is called _____ end feel.

2. A cushioned limitation where soft tissue prevents further movement, such as knee or elbow flexion, is called _____ end feel.

3. It is called _____ end feel, when the limitation is caused by the stretch of fibrous tissue as the joint reaches the extent of its range of motion.

4. Normal end feel happens at the _____ of a normal range of motion and is _____.

5. Sudden pain during passive movement before the end of normal range of motion was termed _____ by Cyriax.

6. Abnormal end feel is indicated during passive movement when there is _____ or _____ in the movement.

7. Passive movement assessment indicates the condition of the _____ tissues.

8. Full, painless passive range of motion indicates that the joint and associated structures are _____.

9. Two indicators of dysfunction are _____ and _____.

10. Resisted or isometric movement is used to assess the condition of the _____ tissues.

11. Indicators of lesions or dysfunction in the contractile tissue are _____ and _____.

12. Another name for resisted or isometric movement assessment is _____.

13. Sensing the difference in tissue quality and integrity through touch is termed _____.

14. A common palpable condition found in muscle that is usually associated with a lesion is a fibrous or _____ band.

15. Examining the outcome of the process in relation to the expected objectives is called _____.

True or False: If the following statements are true, write *true* in the space provided. If they are false, replace the italicized word with one that makes the statement true.

_____ 1. Palpation is most effective when used in conjunction with and *before* assessing range of motion.

_____ 2. When *passive* movement and resisted movement both give positive results, contractile tissues are involved.

_____ 3. A *strong* and painful muscle test indicates a lesion in the inert tissue, possibly a torn ligament or fracture.

_____ 4. The more severe the condition, the more severe the *pain*.

_____ 5. *Taut bands* usually contain trigger points.

Short Answer: Provide short answers to the following questions. Write your answers in the space provided.

1. What information is used in developing session strategies?

   _____

   _____

2. What takes place during the performance phase of the therapeutic procedure?

   _____

   _____

Face and Scalp Massage

Completion: In the space provided, write the word or words that correctly complete each statement.

1. A professional who specializes in facials and skin care is called an _____.

2. The first important step in a face massage is _____ the face.

3. The five classifications of manipulations used for face massage are _____, _____, _____, _____, and _____.

Short Answer: Provide short answers to the following questions. Write your answers in the space provided.

1. When is it determined whether or not to give a face massage?

   _____

2. What products are used for cleansing the face before a massage?

   a. _____

   b. _____

   c. _____

   d. _____

3. What amount of cleansing cream or lotion is used to cleanse the face?

   _____

4. What is used to remove the cleansing product from the face?

   _____

5. Generally, in what direction are the strokes made when removing the cleansing product?

   _____

Short Answer: Provide short answers to the following questions. Write your answers in the space provided.

1. When giving a scalp massage, in what direction are the strokes applied?

   _____

2. What precaution should be observed during scalp massage?

   _____

3. When should scalp massage be avoided?

   _____

Hydrotherapy

Completion: In the space provided, write the word or words that correctly complete each statement.

1. Overexposure to the sun is dangerous to the skin because _____ penetrate the epidermis and affect the living cells of the _____.

2. The skin's main defense against too much sun is to _____.

3. Tanning occurs when ultraviolet rays react with _____ and cause it to darken.

4. One of the primary causes of skin cancer is _____.

5. The sun reacts with the skin to produce vitamin _____.

6. Ultraviolet light therapy is an accepted treatment for the skin condition known as _____.

Completion: In the space provided, write the word or words that correctly complete each statement.

1. The use of heat and cold is a powerful therapeutic agent because the physiological effects are _____.

2. The short application of cold is _____ while prolonged application of cold _____ metabolic activity.

3. The local application of heat causes the blood vessels to _____ and circulation to _____.

4. The application of heat causes the pulse rate to _____ and the white blood cell count to _____.

5. A generalized lowering of the body temperature is termed _____.

Key Choices: The following is a list of reactions to hydrotherapy. Put the appropriate letter(s) in the spaces provided for each of the following conditions.

        C = Cold Application

        H = Heat Application

_____ 1. hypothermia

_____ 2. vasodilation

_____ 3. reduced circulation

_____ 4. anesthetic effect

_____ 5. increased circulation

_____ 6. increased perspiration

_____ 7. numbness

_____ 8. increased white cell count

_____ 9. local muscle relaxation

_____ 10. analgesia

_____ 11. depressed metabolic activity

_____ 12. reduced nerve sensitivity

_____ 13. hyperthermia

_____ 14. decreased muscle spasticity

_____ 15. leukocyte migration into the area

True or False: If the following statements are true, write *true* in the space provided. If they are false, replace the italicized word with one that makes the statement true.

_____ 1. People with very *thin* skin are more prone to spotting, freckling, and skin cancer.

_____ 2. When heat or cold is applied to the body, certain *physiological* changes occur.

_____ 3. A *short* application of cold sedates metabolic activity.

_____ 4. The warming effect of the sun is due to *ultraviolet* rays.

_____ 5. The application of *cold* to a fresh soft-tissue injury will reduce pain and swelling.

Completion: In the space provided, write the word or words that correctly complete each statement.

1. When a body part is submerged in water, it is called a(n) _____.

2. The application of cold agents for therapeutic purposes is termed _____.

3. The application of water to the body for therapeutic purposes is known as _____.

4. The changes produced by water that is above or below body temperature are considered to be _____ effects.

5. The upper temperature limit for water that is considered safe for therapeutic purposes is _____.

6. The normal temperature of the body is _____ or _____.

7. The body's normal skin surface temperature is approximately _____.

8. A bath where only the hips and pelvis is submerged is called a _____.

Short answer: Provide short answers to the following questions. Write your answers in the space provided.

1. List four variables that determine the nature and extent of the effects of heat or cold on the body.

    a. _____

    b. _____

    c. _____

    d. _____

2. What are the three forms in which water is used for therapeutic purposes?

    a. _____

    b. _____

    c. _____

3. What are the properties of water that make it a valuable therapeutic agent?

    a. _____

    b. _____

    c. _____

4. The three classifications of therapeutic effects of water on the body are:

    a. _____

    b. _____

    c. _____

5. List three ways of applying moist heat.

    a. _____

    b. _____

    c. _____

6. The acronym RICE stands for

   a. _____

   b. _____

   c. _____

   d. _____

7. List three economical methods of applying local cold therapy.

   a. _____

   b. _____

   c. _____

8. List the three normal reactions to ice therapy in the order in which they occur.

   a. _____

   b. _____

   c. _____

9. Baths can be classified according to the temperature of the water. What is the temperature range for the following baths?

   a. cold bath — _____ to _____°F

   b. tepid bath — _____ to _____°F

   c. warm bath — _____ to _____°F

   d. hot bath — _____ to _____°F

   e. steam bath — _____ to _____°F

Massage for Nursing and Healthcare

Short Answer: Provide short answers to the following questions. Write your answers in the space provided.

1. What massage system is most frequently used in nursing?

   _____

2. What basic manipulations are most frequently used in nursing?

   _____

3. What is the general goal of using massage in nursing and healthcare?

   _____

4. What is the main difference between nurses who use massage and massage practitioners?

   _____

   _____

   _____

Short Answer: Provide short answers to the following questions. Write your answers in the space provided.

1. List at least two ways that massage benefits the skin.

   a. _____

   b. _____

2. List three ways that massage benefits the muscular system.

   a. _____

   b. _____

   c. _____

3. List three ways that massage benefits the nervous system.

   a. _____

   b. _____

   c. _____

   d. _____

   e. _____

4. List at least three ways that massage benefits the circulatory system.

   a. _____

   b. _____

   c. _____

   d. _____

   e. _____

Short Answer: Provide short answers to the following questions. Write your answers in the space provided.

1. In what direction are effleurage movements given?

   _____

2. What does it mean that effleurage strokes are centripetal?

   _____

3. Manipulations involving the movement of the superficial tissues over or against the deeper tissues are called _____.

4. What preliminary precautions should be taken when massage is administered in cases where there is injury or illness?

   _____

5. What are seven warning signs of cancer?

   a. _____

   b. _____

   c. _____

   d. _____

   e. _____

   f. _____

   g. _____

6. When a massage is given to a person in a hospital bed, what are two adjustments that can be made to improve the delivery of the massage?

a. _____

b. _____

Athletic/Sports Massage

Completion: In the space provided, write the word or words that correctly complete each statement.

1. The 1972 Olympic gold medalist, who was known as "the flying Finn," and who credited daily massage for his success was _____.

2. The application of massage techniques that combine sound anatomical and physiological knowledge, an understanding of strength training and conditioning, and specific massage skills to enhance athletic performance is termed _____ or _____ _____.

3. The study of body movement is termed _____.

4. In sports physiology the _____ principle states that in order to improve either strength or endurance, appropriate stresses must be applied to the system.

5. If the intensity of the athletic training exceeds the body's ability to recuperate, the result will probably be _____.

6. The rhythmic pumping massage manipulation that is applied to the belly of the muscle is called _____.

7. Increasing the amount of blood available in a body area is called _____.

8. If pressure on a tender point causes pain to radiate or refer to another area of the body, that point is considered a _____.

9. The massage technique most often used on trigger points is _____.

10. The amount of pressure a therapist uses on a trigger point is determined by the _____.

11. _____ is applied by rubbing across the fibers of the tendon, muscle, or ligament at a 90° angle to the fibers.

12. The British osteopath who popularized cross fiber friction is _____.

Short Answer: Provide short answers to the following questions. Write your answers in the space provided.

1. Why does athletic massage enable athletes to participate more often in rigorous physical training and conditioning?

   _____

2. How does athletic massage reduce the chance of injury?

   _____

3. List four negative effects of exercise.

   a. _____

   b. _____

   c. _____

   d. _____

4. How long does it normally take for a muscle that has been stressed to the point of fatigue to recuperate?

   _____

5. What are two important effects of compression strokes?

   a. _____

   b. _____

6. In what direction is cross fiber friction given?

   _____

7. How long is a cross fiber stroke?

   _____

   _____

8. What does the acronym PNF stand for?

   _____

Key Choices: Choose the massage technique that best fits the description or is most likely to produce the following effects. Write the appropriate letter next to the description or effect.

A. compression   C. cross fiber friction

B. deep pressure   D. active joint movement

_____ 1. softens adhesions in fibrous tissue

_____ 2. causes increased amounts of blood to remain in the muscle over an extended period of time

_____ 3. reduces fibrosis

_____ 4. adopted from proprioceptive neuromuscular facilitation

_____ 5. rubbing across the fibers of the tendon, muscle, or ligament

_____ 6. used effectively to treat tender points

_____ 7. A rhythmic pumping action to the belly of the muscle

_____ 8. therapist supports the body part in position while the client contracts his or her muscles

_____ 9. promotes increased circulation deep in the muscle

_____ 10. reducing the crystalline roughness that forms between tendons and their sheaths

_____ 11. helps to counteract muscle spasm, improve flexibility, and restore muscle strength

_____ 12. creates hyperemia in the muscle tissue

_____ 13. deactivates trigger points and increases function to the referred area

_____ 14. based on Sherington's physiological principles

_____ 15. stretches, broadens and separates muscle fibers

_____ 16. encourages the formation of strong, pliable scar tissue at the sight of healing injuries

_____ 17. based on reciprocal inhibition and post-isometric relaxation

Key Choices: Choose the athletic massage application that best fits the description. Write the letter of the application next to the description in the space provided.

     A = Post-event massage

     B = Pre-event massage

     C = Rehabilitative massage

     D = Restorative massage

_____ 1. focuses on the restoration of tissue function following injury

_____ 2. given within the first hour or two after participating in an event

_____ 3. breaks down transverse adhesions that may have resulted from previous injuries

_____ 4. warms and loosens the muscles causing hyperemia in specific muscle areas

_____ 5. can locate and relieve areas of stress that carry a high risk of injury

_____ 6. stimulates circulation and at the same time calms the nervous system

_____ 7. reduces fibrosis caused by muscle injury

_____ 8. given 15 to 45 minutes prior to an event

_____ 9. is considered a regular and valuable part of the athlete's training schedule

_____ 10. enables the athlete to reach his or her peak performance earlier in the event and maintain that performance longer

_____ 11. allows the athlete to train at a higher level of intensity, more consistently with less chance of injury

_____ 12. three to four times as effective as rest in recovery from muscle fatigue

_____ 13. shortens the time it takes for an injury to heal

_____ 14. makes more intense and frequent workouts possible, thereby improving overall performance

_____ 15. prevents delayed onset of muscle soreness and reduces the time it takes for the body to recover from exertion

_____ 16. is fast paced and invigorating

_____ 17. accelerates healing so the athlete's "down time" is cut to a minimum

_____ 18. helps to form strong, pliable scar tissue

_____ 19. given after the athlete has had a chance to warm down from the exertion of the competition or exercise

True or False: If the following statements are true, write *true* in the space provided. If they are false, replace the italicized word with one that makes the statement true.

_____ 1. Pre-event massage increases flexibility and circulation and *replaces* the warm up before an event.

_____ 2. During *pre-event massage,* adhesions can be eliminated to reduce the chance of injury.

_____ 3. Post-event massage is given after competition and helps an athlete *cool down.*

_____ 4. *Post-event massage* is three to four times as effective as rest in recovery from muscle fatigue.

_____ 5. *Restorative massage* may resemble pre-event or post-event massage.

_____ 6. A *strain* involves the stretching or tearing of a ligament.

_____ 7. A *grade I* strain is the most severe.

_____ 8. As a muscle fiber contracts, the sarcolemma and the *endomysium* move as a unit.

Short Answer: Provide short answers to the following questions. Write your answers in the space provided.

1. What is the first step when giving a post-event massage?

   _____

2. After a long race, what are some conditions the therapist needs to watch for?

   _____

3. What action should the therapist take if strains, sprains, abrasions, or contusions are apparent?

   _____

4. When interviewing an athlete for determining a training massage program, what are five important questions to ask?

   a. _____

   b. _____

   c. _____

   d. _____

   e. _____

Completion: In the space provided, write the word or words that correctly complete each statement.

1. Athletic injuries that have a sudden and definite onset and are usually of relatively short duration are considered to be _____ injuries.

2. A muscle strain in which there is severe tearing and complete loss of function is called a grade _____ strain.

3. The therapist's indicator as to how intensely to work on an injury site is _____.

4. Athletic injuries that have a gradual onset, tend to last for a long time, or reoccur often are considered _____ injuries.

Short Answer: Provide short answers to the following questions. Write your answers in the space provided.

1. Give six examples of acute athletic injuries.

    a. _____   b. _____

    c. _____   d. _____

    e. _____   f. _____

2. What effect does RICE have on soft tissue injuries?

    _____

3. When can massage be started on injured tissue?

    _____

4. What are two goals the therapist strives to achieve when working on chronic conditions?

    a. _____

    b. _____

5. List two positive effects of the swelling that results from tissue damage.

    a. _____

    b. _____

6. List two negative effects of swelling that results from tissue damage.

    a. _____

    b. _____

    c. _____

Key Choices: Identify the following conditions as either chronic or acute. Write the appropriate letter next to the conditions described below.

C = Chronic

A = Acute

_____ 1. dislocated shoulder

_____ 2. iliotibial band syndrome

_____ 3. shin splints

_____ 4. broken wrist

_____ 5. overuse syndrome

_____ 6. torn ligament

_____ 7. sprained ankle

_____ 8. tennis elbow

_____ 9. bruised hip

_____ 10. tendonitis

Completion: In the space provided, write the word or words that correctly complete each statement.

1. The tensile strength of connective tissue is provided by _____.

2. The layer of connective tissue that closely covers an individual muscle is the _____.

3. Connective tissue extends beyond the end of the muscle to become _____.

4. The perimysium extends inward from the epimysium and separates the muscle into bundles of muscle fibers or _____.

5. Each muscle fiber is covered by a delicate connective tissue covering called the _____.

6. Soft tissue injuries result in the tearing of _____ in the connective tissue.

7. Collagen fibers are produced by _____.

8. Collagen formation that reconnects the injured tissue forms _____.

9. Collagen fibers that connect to structures other than the injured tissue form _____ that restrict mobility.

10. Proper _____ reduces the degree of secondary trauma following soft tissue injury.

Specialized Massage

Completion: In the space provided, write the word or words that correctly complete each statement.

1. The massage practitioner can sharpen his or her skills and stay current to new developments in the massage field through _____.

2. Massage given to a pregnant woman is commonly called _____.

3. The main goal of prenatal massage is _____.

Short Answer: Provide short answers to the following questions. Write your answers in the space provided.

1. What are two considerations when positioning a pregnant woman for massage?

   a. _____

   b. _____

2. Why is the supine position not recommended during the later stages of pregnancy?

   _____

3. What is the major general contraindication for massage during pregnancy?

   _____

Completion: In the space provided, write the word or words that correctly complete each statement.

1. The Dane credited with developing manual lymph drainage massage was

   _____.

2. Thin-walled tubes that collect lymph from interstitial fluid in the tissues are called

   _____.

3. White blood cells produced in the lymph system are known as _____.

4. Small bean-shaped masses of lymphatic tissue located along the course of lymph vessels are termed _____.

5. The principle manipulations used in lymph massage are _____ and

   _____.

Short Answer: Provide short answers to the following questions. Write your answers in the space provided.

1. Where does lymph re-enter the blood stream?

   _____

2. What portion of the interstitial fluid that is reabsorbed into the circulatory system becomes lymph?

   _____

3. What causes lymph to move through the system?

   _____

   _____

4. The two main functions of lymph nodes are:

   a. _____

   b. _____

5. What kind of massage is applied to neurolymphatic reflexes?

   _____

6. In what direction is lymph massage given?

   _____

7. When doing lymph massage on the leg, where should the manipulations begin?

   _____

Completion: In the space provided, write the word or words that correctly complete each statement.

1. Massage styles that are directed toward the deeper tissue structures of the muscle and fascia are commonly called _____ massage.

2. Rolfing was developed by _____.

3. Neurophysiological therapies recognize the link between the _____ system and the _____ system.

4. Alterations or disturbances in the neuromuscular relationship often result in _____ and _____.

5. A hyperirritable spot that is painful when compressed is called a _____.

6. When a point is compressed and it refers pain to another area of the body, that point is considered an _____.

7. If a point is hypersensitive when compressed but does not refer pain, it is considered a _____.

8. The technique used by massage therapists where direct pressure is applied to the trigger point is known as _____.

Short Answer: Provide short answers to the following questions. Write your answers in the space provided.

1. What are three types of neuro-physiological therapies?

   a. _____

   b. _____

   c. _____

2. Where are myofascial trigger points found?

   _____

3. What is the neurological phenomenon that links a trigger point to its associated dysfunctional tissue?

   _____

4. How are taut bands of muscle located?

   _____

5. What are three common areas associated with the muscle where trigger points are found?

   a. _____

   b. _____

   c. _____

6. List four common procedures for deactivating trigger points.

   a. _____

   b. _____

   c. _____

   d. _____

7. What is the regulating factor in determining how much pressure to use when deactivating trigger points?

   _____

8. When a trigger point has been released, what action should be taken on the muscle where it was located?

   _____

Short Answer: Provide short answers to the following questions. Write your answers in the space provided.

1. Who originally developed Neuromuscular Therapy in the 1930s?

   _____

2. What are common abnormal signs associated with neuromuscular lesions?

   a. _____

   b. _____

   c. _____

   d. _____

   e. _____

   f. _____

   g. _____

   h. _____

   i. _____

3. Besides trigger points, what other areas does Neuromuscular Therapy (NMT) recognize that may be tender when palpated?

   _____

4. The main massage manipulations used in NMT are:

   a. _____

   b. _____

   c. _____

   d. _____

Completion: In the space provided, write the word or words that correctly complete each statement.

1. A therapeutic procedure that is used to improve the functional mobility of the joints and goes by the acronym MET is _____.

2. The two basic inhibitory reflexes produced during MET manipulations are _____ _____ and _____.

Short Answer: Provide short answers to the following questions. Write your answers in the space provided.

1. The three main variations of MET are:

   a. _____

   b. _____

   c. _____

2. Which of the three variations of MET use post-isometric relaxation?

_____

3. Which of the three variations of MET use reciprocal inhibition?

_____

4. What conditions respond best to MET?

_____

Short Answer: Provide short answers to the following questions. Write your answers in the space provided.

1. The gentlest of soft tissue manipulations when addressing mobility restrictions due to pain and soft tissue dysfunction are _____.

2. Three body-work systems that incorporate this technique are:

    a. _____

    b. _____

    c. _____

3. What is the difference between these three techniques?

    _____

4. Strain-counterstrain (tender point) technique was developed by _____.

5. What is the main treatment in strain counterstrain?

    _____

    _____

    _____

6. Orthobionomy was developed by an English osteopath named _____.

7. The hands-on manipulations used in orthobionomy are _____ and _____.

8. The main physical techniques used in structural muscular balancing include:

    a. _____

    b. _____

    c. _____

    d. _____

9. What are the two main goals of structural muscular balancing?

   a. _____

   b. _____

Completion: In the space provided, write the word or words that correctly complete each statement.

1. A traditional Chinese medical practice whereby the skin is punctured with needles at specific points for therapeutic purposes is known as _____.

2. Religious philosophies of the Far East speak of _____ or "the way" or "that which is all there is."

3. In eastern philosophies the opposing yet complementary aspects of existence are represented by _____ and _____.

Matching: Arrange the following words in two columns. In the first column, list words that correspond to *yin*. In the second column, write the words that correspond to *yang* adjacent to the contrasting word in the *yin* column.

active	back of the body	cold	contracting
dark	day	deficient	excessive
expanding	forceful	front of the body	high
hot	inner body	inside	light
low	lower body	night	outer body
outside	overactive	passive	underactive
upper body	weak		

YIN   **YANG**

_____   _____

_____   _____

_____   _____

_____   _____

_____   _____

_____   _____

_____   _____

_____   _____

_____   _____

_____   _____

_____   _____

_____   _____

Completion: In the space provided, write the word or words that correctly complete each statement.

1.   The interaction of yin and yang creates a vibratory force or energy called _____.

2.   In the human body, there are three sources of this vital force. They are:

    a. _____

    b. _____

    c. _____

3.   According to ancient philosophy, this vital force manifests itself as five interrelated elements. They are:

    a. _____   d. _____

    b. _____   e. _____

    c. _____

4.   Chi moves through the body in specific channels called _____.

5.   There are _____ bilateral channels that relate to the organs.

6.   Along these channels are small areas of high conductivity called

    _____.

7.   A number of treatment systems that incorporate various manipulations (not needles) on acupoints are collectively called _____.

8.   The Japanese system of finger pressure massage is called _____.

9.   The art and science of stimulating certain points on the body (especially the hands and feet) that effect organs or functions in distant parts of the body is known as _____.

Therapeutic Exercise

Completion: In the space provided, write the word or words that correctly complete each statement.

1. Exercise that is done with the intent of improving some physical condition is considered _____.

2. The principle of applying stresses to the body greater than it is accustomed to in order to cause physiological change is known as the _____ principle.

3. The body changes to tolerate the increased load through the process of _____.

4. The ability of a muscle or muscle group to contract and produce tension with a force exerted on some resistance is called _____.

5. The strength of a muscle is measured by _____.

6. The increased bulk of a muscle and increased density of the capillary bed within the muscle is called _____.

7. The muscle fibers controlled by a single motor neuron are collectively called a _____.

8. In order for adaptive increases in strength to occur, the muscles must contract against a force that is at least _____ percent of the maximum capacity.

9. In order to increase muscle function, the muscle must be exercised to a point of _____.

10. Maximum resistance with low reps tend to build muscle _____ and _____.

11. Lighter resistance with high repetitions builds muscle _____.

Short Answer: Provide short answers to the following questions. Write your answers in the space provided.

1. Before suggesting an exercise to a client, what must the therapist know:

   a. about the exercise?

   _____

   b. about the client?

   _____

2.   What is the goal of therapeutic exercise?

_____

3.   List five physiological areas that can be improved through therapeutic exercise.

   a. _____

   b. _____

   c. _____

   d. _____

   e. _____

4.   List four factors that determine the relative strength of a muscle.

   a. _____

   b. _____

   c. _____

   d. _____

5.   What is the main disadvantage of isometric strengthening exercises?

_____

6.   List three possible sources of resistance for isotonic exercises.

   a. _____

   b. _____

   c. _____

True or False: If the following statements are true, write *true* in the space provided. If they are false, replace the italicized word with one that makes the statement true.

_____   1.   The increased bulk of a muscle is the result of an increase in the thickness of the *actin and myosin filaments*.

_____   2.   The larger the cross sectional size of the muscle, the greater the *endurance*.

_____   3.   Most *strengthening* exercises increase muscle strength and endurance.

_____   4.   A maximum isometric contraction will generate approximately 20 percent more force than a maximum *eccentric* contraction.

_____   5.   During isotonic exercises, eccentric contractions should be *slower* than concentric contractions for maximum benefit.

_____   6.   As a muscle contracts through its available range of motion, the *force* it generates varies.

Key Choices: Choose the types of muscle contractions that best fit the descriptions or are most likely to produce the following effects. Write the appropriate letter next to the stated description or effect in the space provided.

A. concentric contraction   C. isometric contraction

B. eccentric contraction   D. isotonic contraction

_____ 1. Movement occurs.

_____ 2. The muscle length remains the same.

_____ 3. The muscle lengthens during the contraction.

_____ 4. The force of the contraction is different than the resistance.

_____ 5. The force of the contraction is equal to the resistance.

_____ 6. The force of contraction is greater than the resistance.

_____ 7. There is no perceivable movement.

_____ 8. The muscle shortens during the contraction.

_____ 9. The force of the contraction is less than the resistance.

Completion: In the space provided, write the word or words that correctly complete each statement.

1. Exercises that provide a maximum load at several points during a muscle contraction are _____ exercises.

2. During manual resistance exercises, resistance is provided by _____ _____.

3. The direction of the resistance in manual resistance exercises is _____ _____.

4. The point of therapist contact in manual resistance exercises is _____ _____.

5. Body weight exercises use _____ to supply the resistance.

6. Push-ups and pull-ups are examples of _____ exercises.

7. The ability to carry on an activity over a prolonged period of time and resist fatigue is called _____.

8. Two body systems affected by endurance training are the _____ and _____ systems.

9. General endurance is sometimes called _____ endurance.

10. The ability of an individual to continue a general exercise over an extended period of time is called _____.

11. General endurance can be improved with regular _____.

12. The amount of stress or overload put on the cardiovascular system by aerobic exercise is related to the _____ of the exercise.

Short Answer: Provide short answers to the following questions. Write your answers in the space provided.

1. What are two advantages to body weight exercises?

    a. _____

    b. _____

2. List three examples of mechanical resistance equipment.

    a. _____

    b. _____

    c. _____

3. List four factors that determine the effectiveness of aerobic exercise.

    a. _____

    b. _____

    c. _____

    d. _____

4. Name four pieces of mechanical exercise equipment that are designed to improve cardiovascular fitness.

    a. _____

    b. _____

    c. _____

    d. _____

5. List at least seven aerobic activities.

    a. _____ e. _____

    b. _____ f. _____

    c. _____ g. _____

    d. _____

6. What is the recommended frequency for aerobic exercise to maintain cardiorespiratory fitness?

    _____

7. What is the formula for determining a person's maximum heart rate?

    _____

8. According to the American College of Sports Medicine, at what intensity are the optimum benefits of cardiovascular training obtained?

   _____

   _____

9. Determine the high and low heart rate limit for cardiopulmonary benefit for an individual thirty-two years of age.

   a. _____

   b. _____

10. List the three basic components of an aerobic workout.

   a. _____

   b. _____

   c. _____

11. List five physiological adaptations that result from regular aerobic exercise.

   a. _____

   b. _____

   c. _____

   d. _____

   e. _____

12. List six benefits of cardiorespiratory fitness.

   a. _____

   b. _____

   c. _____

   d. _____

   e. _____

   f. _____

13. List five factors that may result in reduced flexibility.

   a. _____

   b. _____

   c. _____

   d. _____

   e. _____

14. What are two physiological changes that take place that allow elongation of muscle tissue.

a. _____

b. _____

Completion: In the space provided, write the word or words that correctly complete each statement.

1. The ability of a joint to move freely and painlessly through its range of motion is called _____.

2. When decreased extensibility of muscle or other tissues crossing the joint causes reduced joint mobility, it is termed a _____.

3. The ability of tissue to return to normal resting length when stress is removed from it is called _____.

4. The property that allows tissues to change shape and adapt to ongoing stresses and conditions is termed _____.

5. Exercises that move the affected segment of the body through its available movement are called _____.

6. If the body segment is moved by some external force without the voluntary contractions of the muscles acting upon that segment, it is called _____.

7. The type of manipulation used to determine where limitations of movement exist but does not challenge those limitations is called _____.

8. Range of motion done by an individual voluntarily contracting muscles is called _____ range of motion.

9. Elongating of soft tissue in order to maintain or increase full range of motion is accomplished with _____.

10. The sensory receptors responsible for the myotatic reflex are the _____ and the _____.

11. Sensory organs, located in the muscles, that monitor the velocity and extent of muscle movement are called _____.

12. Sensory organs, located near musculotendinous junctions, that monitor tension are the _____.

13. The myotatic reflex is initiated when _____ and causes _____.

14. _____ stretching moves a body segment beyond its free range of motion, while the muscles that act on that segment remain relaxed.

15. In _____ stretching, another person or therapist moves the client's body into the stretching positions, while the client remains relaxed.

16. Stretching techniques that utilize neuromuscular reflexes to enhance the elongation of muscles are referred to as _____ stretches.

17. When a muscle acting on a joint contracts and the muscle that causes the opposite action is reflexively inhibited, the physiological process is called _____

18. The complex neuromuscular process of using the correct sequence of muscular movements with the right timing and force is referred to as _____.

19. Improving skill and coordination requires _____ and _____.

20. The relationship and alignment of body parts usually observed in the standing position is referred to as _____.

21. When the body is balanced between left and right, back and front, and the segments of the axial skeleton are properly aligned, a person is said to have _____.

True or False: If the following statements are true, write *true* in the space provided. If they are false, replace the italicized word with one that makes the statement true.

_____ 1. The *plastic* property of fibrous tissue regulates its flexibility.

_____ 2. Range of motion exercises are effective for *increasing* flexibility.

_____ 3. *Ballistic* stretches suppress the stretch reflex and inhibit the GTO.

_____ 4. The *Golgi tendon organs,* located in the muscle belly, sense the extent of muscle movement.

_____ 5. *Expiration* takes place because of the contraction of the diaphragm.

Short Answer: Provide short answers to the following questions. Write your answers in the space provided.

1. How much force is used in manual passive stretching exercises?

_____

2. What four aspects of a manual passive stretch does the therapist control?

a. _____

b. _____

c. _____

d. _____

3. What are three variations of the reflexive inhibition stretching technique?

a. _____

b. _____

c. _____

4. Name three sets of auxiliary muscles that assist during deep inhalation.

   a. _____

   b. _____

   c. _____

5. Why is it important to breath through the nose instead of the mouth?

   _____

Massage Business Administration

Business Practices

Short Answer: Provide short answers to the following questions. Write your answers in the space provided.

1. When does business planning begin?

   _____

2. When does business planning end?

   _____

3. Name four important parts of business planning.

   a. _____

   b. _____

   c. _____

   d. _____

4. What are three common types of business operations?

   a. _____

   b. _____

   c. _____

Completion: In the space provided, write the word or words that correctly complete each statement.

1. A short general statement of the main focus of the business is called the

   _____.

2. Specific, attainable, measurable things or accomplishments that you set and make a commitment to achieve are termed _____.

3. If you are an individual owner of a business and carry all expenses, obligations, liabilities, and assets, you are considered a _____.

4. In order to establish a _____, a charter must be obtained from the state in which the business operates.

5. Management of a corporation is carried on by a _____.

6. When beginning a business, the expenses incurred before any revenues are collected are considered _____.

7. Two primary reasons for the failure of small businesses are _____ and _____.

Short Answer: Provide short answers to the following questions. Write your answers in the space provided.

1. If your business is a sole proprietorship, who is responsible for any debts, losses or debts?

    _____

2. What zoning requirements must be considered when choosing a massage business location?

    _____

3. List at least two important considerations when buying an established business.

    a. _____

    b. _____

    c. _____

Completion: In the space provided, write the word or words that correctly complete each statement.

1. If a business is operating under a name other than the owner's, a _____ _____ is required.

2. If the business sells products or if services are taxed, a _____ must be obtained from _____.

3. To assure the business meets zoning requirements, the _____ _____ should be contacted.

4. An Employer Identification Number (EIN) must be obtained from the _____ if the business hires employees.

5. The identification number issued to licensed healthcare providers and used when submitting claims to medical insurance companies is called a _____.

6. As a massage business owner, one should have adequate insurance against _____, _____, and _____.

Key Choices: Choose the types of insurance that best fits the description. Write the appropriate letter next to the stated description in the space provided.

A. automobile insurance

B. disability insurance

C. fire and theft insurance

D. health insurance

E. liability insurance

F. malpractice insurance

G. workers' compensation insurance

_____ 1. protects the individual from loss of income because they are unable to work due to long-term illness or injury

_____ 2. helps cover the cost of medical bills, especially hospitalization, serious injury, or illness

_____ 3. provides medical and liability insurance to the driver and any passengers

_____ 4. is required if you have employees

_____ 5. covers the cost of fixtures, furniture, equipment, products, and supplies

_____ 6. covers costs of injuries and litigation resulting from injuries sustained on the owner's property

_____ 7. covers the medical costs for the employee if they are injured on the job

_____ 8. covers the vehicle and its contents, regardless of who is at fault

_____ 9. protects the therapist from lawsuits filed by a client because of injury or loss that results from negligence or substandard performance

Completion: In the space provided, write the word or words that correctly complete each statement.

1. The standards of acceptable and professional behavior by which a person or business conducts business are called _____.

2. When setting your fees for massage, the _____ and the _____ should be considered.

3. A summary of all sales and cash receipts is called an _____.

4. A ledger that records, separates, and classifies business expenditures is called a _____.

Short Answer: Provide short answers to the following questions. Write your answers in the space provided.

1. If a massage business is operated out of a home, are all telephone expenses tax deductible?

_____

2. For a self-employed massage practitioner, what three major records should be maintained?

a. _____

b. _____

c. _____

3. Two important reasons for keeping accurate financial records are:

    a. _____

    b. _____

4. Why is it advisable to consult an accountant when preparing taxes?

    _____

    _____

5. What name is on the business checking account?

    _____

6. What moneys are deposited in the business account?

    _____

7. For what purposes are checks written from the business account?

    _____

8. What is the purpose of a petty cash fund?

    _____

9. Where does petty cash fund money come from?

    _____

10. How long should canceled checks and bank statements be kept for tax purposes?

    _____

11. What is included in the income records?

    _____

12. Name ten things that should be included on an income receipt or invoice.

    a. _____   f. _____

    b. _____   g. _____

    c. _____   h. _____

    d. _____   i. _____

    e. _____   j. _____

13. How many copies of the invoice should there be and where do they go?

_____

14. Information that is included in each entry of the disbursement ledger includes:

   a. _____

   b. _____

   c. _____

   d. _____

   e. _____

15. What receipts should be kept and filed?

_____

16. How long should receipts be kept?

_____

17. When is it necessary to keep an accounts receivable file?

_____

18. A record of money owed to other persons or businesses is kept in an _____ file.

19. Items and equipment purchased to be used in the business for an extended period of time [more than a year] are called _____.

20. Are the products that are for sale in the business considered business assets?

_____

21. What information should be kept in a record of business assets?

_____

_____

22. What are two methods of determining business-related automobile expenses?

_____

23. What is usually kept in a client record?

    a. _____

    b. _____

    c. _____

24. What is the importance of an appointment book?

    _____

    _____

Completion: In the space provided, write the word or words that correctly complete each statement.

1. The business activity done to promote and increase business is called _____.

2. A segment of the population with similar characteristics that the practitioner may prefer to attract is his or her _____.

3. Most promotional activities are _____ in nature.

4. Any marketing activity that the practitioner must pay for directly is considered _____.

5. The practice of encouraging clients to come back for services repeatedly is known as _____.

Short Answer: Provide short answers to the following questions. Write your answers in the space provided.

1. List five marketing activities.

    a. _____

    b. _____

    c. _____

    d. _____

    e. _____

2. What is the advantage of selecting a target market?

    _____

    _____

3. What are two ways of determining a target market?

    a. _____

    b. _____

    _____

4. What are two objectives of promotional activities?

    a. _____

    b. _____

5. Give three examples of promotional activities.

    a. _____

    b. _____

    c. _____

6. Give four examples of promotional materials.

    a. _____

    b. _____

    c. _____

    d. _____

7. What should be included on every piece of promotional material?

    _____

8. List four ways to promote business through public relations.

    a. _____

    b. _____

    c. _____

    d. _____

9. What are two main sources for obtaining referrals?

    a. _____

    b. _____

10. When a satisfied client refers a new person, what should be done?

    _____

11. When a healthcare professional refers a client, what should be done?

    a. _____

    b. _____

    c. _____

12. What are the three "R's" of referrals?

a. _____

b. _____

c. _____

Short Answer: Provide short answers to the following questions. Write your answers in the space provided.

1. What federal regulations must be observed when operating a massage business with employees?

a. _____

b. _____

c. _____

2. What state regulations must be observed when operating a massage business?

a. _____

b. _____

c. _____

d. _____

e. _____